Great Comebacks from Ostomy Surgery

The inspirational stories of 15 people who have survived and thrived following ostomy surgery

by
ROLF BENIRSCHKE
with Elaine Minamide

Rolf Benirschke Enterprises
San Diego, California

Great Comebacks from Ostomy Surgery
by Rolf Benirschke with Elaine Minamide

FIRST EDITION

ISBN 0-9720065-0-8

Cover and back photos: Greg Schneider & Amy Conner

Cover and interior design: Michael Loftus/Loftus Design Associates

Printed in the United States of America

TABLE OF CONTENTS

Great Comebacks from Ostomy Surgery

Dedication

To everyone facing ostomy surgery . . .
and to their family and friends
who help them get through it.

ACKNOWLEDGEMENTS

The writing of *Great Comebacks from Ostomy Surgery* has been a desire of mine ever since I was forced to recover from my own ostomy surgery back in 1979. That was a difficult time for me because I had to reconcile what I believed to be such a cruel and unfair experience for someone of my age to go through. After all, I was young, I was just beginning my career as a professional athlete, and I had always been healthy. This just wasn't supposed to happen.

As I went through my recovery, I learned that there are approximately 130,000 other such surgeries performed each year in the United States. I know that each operation is a life-changing experience for the patient and their family and that everyone goes through the same feelings of anger and frustration and difficulty coming to grips with their situation as I did. I also realize that I was fortunate when I went through my illness to be a part of a professional football team that was loved and supported by the community. Not everyone is so lucky, and many go through their trials alone and with little encouragement from people around them.

Great Comebacks from Ostomy Surgery was written for these people and with the idea that if we could find individuals who everyone—young or old, male or female, athletic or not—could relate to, then we would have a book that delivers a huge impact. With the help of ET nurses around the country, colon and rectal surgeons, and patients I have met over the years, I have assembled a special collection of stories that I believe will become a valuable resource for new patients facing ostomy surgery.

The putting together of *Great Comebacks from Ostomy Surgery* would not have been possible without the support and encouragement from the volunteers at the Crohn's & Colitis Foundation of America, the United Ostomy Association, and the people I have had the good fortune of working with at ConvaTec. Since the company was founded in 1978, ConvaTec's commitment to its patients has been unwavering and has propelled the company into the world leader in the manufacture and distribution of ostomy supplies. I consider it a privilege to speak on their behalf and encourage patients facing ostomy surgery.

Although I am convinced this book will encourage and inspire anyone who reads it, I am reminded that the decision to get "better" and not "bitter" is still up to the patient . . . and it *is* a decision. When I was playing in the NFL, we had top-notch coaches teaching and preparing us for the games we played each week. When Game Day rolled around, however, and the players crossed the "white lines" onto the field, it became up to us. The outcome of the game was determined by how well we performed individually and how well we executed the game plan we had been taught.

And so it is with ostomy surgery. After reading this book, I hope you will come away with the understanding that while our circumstances can seem incredibly difficult and brutally unfair at times, that is life. What becomes important is how we each deal with the situation. In this book, you will read about some remarkable people who have gone through some dreadful medical experiences, but who each made the decision not to let their circumstances control the outcome of their situations.

When we make the same decision we have the opportunity to discover the indomitable human spirit that God has gifted each of us with. We can use these difficult circumstances to completely transform us, and the people around us, and turn our medical situations into one of the greatest blessings of our lives. I know because that happened to me and to each of the people whose stories you are about to read.

I hope you enjoy *Great Comebacks from Ostomy Surgery* and find great inspiration from these individuals who are excited to help show others the way.

Foreword

by Victor Fazio, M.D.

Chairman of the Department of Colon-Rectal Surgery at the Cleveland Clinic

There's a good chance you're holding this book because you're considering an ostomy operation. For well over thirty years, I've met with patients like you, and you're probably wondering if ostomy surgery is all that it's cracked up to be. Will you really be able to do all the things you love to do after the operation, or is this just some sales pitch tossed out by us doctors to get you to submit? What about traveling, participating in sports, getting married, and having children? What about making love?

I've heard all the questions, and I know that the thought of wearing an appliance to collect a person's waste sounds like a fate worse than death. When people make an appointment to see me, they have usually reached the end of the line. They've withstood years of physical discomfort, suffered through long bouts of intestinal distress, and endured embarrassing episodes of incontinence or loss of bowel control. Most have tried everything possible to avoid the surgery, but after all else failed and their lives remained compromised and in danger, they understood that ostomy surgery is their last chance.

It makes me sad to think of what people like you have gone through. Not just you but your families, your kids, your parents, and your friends. Sad because I know it doesn't have to be that way . . . and shouldn't be that way. You see, I have performed more than 5,000 ostomy surgeries since 1973, and the almost universal reaction I receive soon after the operation is, "Doctor, if I had only known I was going to feel this good, I never would have waited so long."

Now, instead of having to convince patients on my own, I can just hand them a copy of *Great Comebacks from Ostomy Surgery*. Finally, we have a resource that can help patients get the answers and be inspired at the same time. With this collection of compelling and true stories about actual patients, Rolf Benirschke demonstrates that you don't have to just survive ostomy surgery, you can actually thrive!

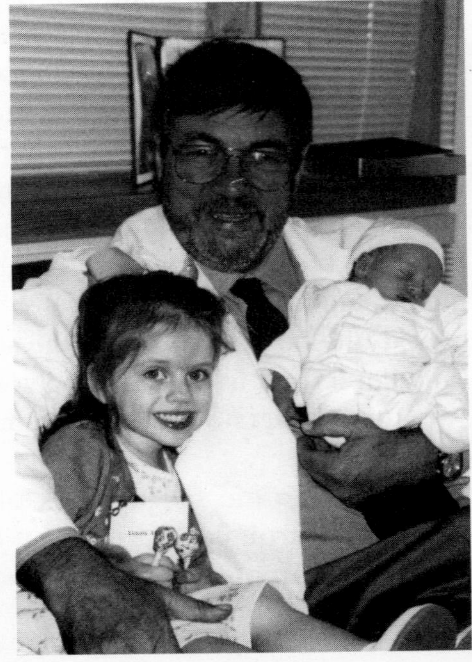

Dr. Vic Fazio cuddles two miracle children: Victoria and Stephen Ambrosi. You'll learn the rest of the story in Lucy Ambrosi's chapter beginning on page 51.

Victor W. Fazio, M.D., is chairman of the Department of Colorectal Surgery and vice-chairman of the Division of Surgery at The Cleveland Clinic in Cleveland, Ohio. He has held both positions for more than twenty years. Board-certified in colon and rectal surgery, Dr. Fazio's clinical interests are Crohn's disease and ulcerative colitis, colorectal cancer, and pelvic floor reservoir procedures for ulcerative colitis and familial polyposis.

Dr. Fazio was awarded the Premier Physician Award from the Crohn's & Colitis Foundation in 1992. Under his co-direction, treatment for digestive diseases at The Cleveland Clinic is ranked second in the country in U.S. News & World Report's *annual survey of top hospitals. In 2000, he was the first recipient of The Cleveland Clinic Master Clinician Award.*

A frequent lecturer at national and international medical meetings, Dr. Fazio has authored more than 500 scientific papers on surgical management of Crohn's disease, ulcerative colitis, and surgical treatment for colorectal cancers, as well as ostomy management. He has also written seven books on what he has learned in the surgical bay over the years.

My Story

ROLF BENIRSCHKE

AGE

47

HOMETOWN

San Diego, California

MEDICAL SITUATION

In his second season as the place-kicker with the San Diego Chargers, Rolf became sick with inflammatory bowel disease and would need life-saving ostomy surgery at the age of twenty-four.

"Rolf, we need to know more. I'm scheduling you for a colonoscopy tomorrow. A visual exam should help us make the diagnosis more conclusive," announced my physician.

The idea that my doctor would insert a long metal instrument up my rectum and into my colon to see whether there was inflammation or ulcerations on the colon's lining sounded painful and perhaps the most humiliating medical test a human being could be asked to endure.

How had it all come to this? I was twenty-four years old, and before the diarrhea and abdominal spasms started, in great health. In fact, I was a professional athlete—the placekicker for the San Diego Chargers. I was in my second season with the team and was earning a reputation as one of the league's most accurate young kickers. For several weeks, however, I had struggled with severe abdominal cramps, bloody diarrhea, and a persistent fever. My doctor initially prescribed Prednisone (a powerful anti-inflammatory corticosteroid drug) and Azulfidine (an anti-bacterial drug), but my condition failed to improve. Suspecting that I might have Crohn's disease, he decided that I needed a colonoscopy to find out for sure.

The day of the procedure was a memorable one. After checking in with the nurse, I was handed a hospital gown, told to change, and then directed to lie face down on the examining table. If you have ever worn one of those gowns, then you know how hard it is to preserve any modesty. I felt as though my backside was open for the whole world to see.

"So, this is what a professional football player looks like," the nurse joked, trying to be clever as she readied me for the procedure. I was in no mood for humor and gritted my teeth until I was given the mild anesthesia. Although I couldn't feel much, I had a vague sensation that I was being "plumbed" by an invasive device traveling up way too far. Let's just say the scoping procedure will never be on my Top Ten list of fun things to do.

Despite the "view" and biopsy, my physicians were unable to confirm a diagnosis other than to say that I had inflammatory bowel disease (IBD). They were fairly confident that I had Crohn's disease but could not rule out ulcerative colitis. I would later learn that almost one million people in the United States suffer from IBD and that approximately 15 percent of those cases can't be conclusively diagnosed either. (I would live under the impression that I had Crohn's disease for four years before finding out that it was ulcerative colitis all along.)

Despite the best efforts of my doctors, my health continued to deteriorate. Although I was able to keep playing during the 1978 NFL football season, I was steadily losing weight and strength. By midseason, I was no longer strong enough to kick off effectively, although I continued to kick field goals and extra points. Things got worse during the last month of the season.

Eating caused terrible pain and horrible cramping each time my severely inflamed gut received food, so I basically stopped eating. I needed nutrition to perform on the football field, however, so my doctors decided that I should be fed intravenously. In this way, my body would receive enough calories while my bowels would receive a rest.

I settled into the following routine: kick during Sunday's game, check into the hospital Sunday night, and have a central total parental nutritional (TPN) line inserted into my jugular vein, from which I would receive "liquid food" all week. On Saturday, I would be released from the hospital to join the team's road trip or spend the night locally at the Charger's team hotel prior to Sunday's home game. Following the final whistle, I would once again check myself into the hospital and get hooked back up to the TPN line. The only physical exercise I was allowed during the week were laps I could make around the hospital halls.

Looking back on all this, I realize how crazy this schedule sounds. But remember, in my mind and to others around me, I had a bad "stomach ache" and a touch of diarrhea. Pro football players learn to play with pain; after all, this was the NFL, where my teammates were separating shoulders, tearing up knees, and sustaining all kinds of other real injuries, yet they continued to play on Game Day.

But there was another motivation to endure the weeklong IVs and hospital stays. I was scared . . . frightened to death. I was scared that the awful pain would never go away. That I would spend the rest of my life knowing where every bathroom was and that I would never be healthy again. My life was flashing before me, and I didn't like what I was seeing.

But mostly, I was scared that I might lose my job. I loved being an NFL kicker. I loved the competition and the fact that people were counting on me. I loved that my kicks often had a big impact on the outcome of a game. Playing in the NFL was exciting, and I didn't want to give it up or let some stupid disease take that experience away from me. You see, in professional football there is room for only one kicker on a team. You were either playing every Sunday, or you were bounced out of the league. I knew that if I were forced to take some time off, I would be replaced and probably lose my job. Those thoughts petrified me, so I endured. I kept my thoughts and fears to myself and carried on . . . trying desperately to make it to the end of the season.

The weird thing was that I continued to kick well. At one point, I hit sixteen consecutive field goals, and under our new coach Don Coryell and quarterback Dan Fouts, the team was really coming together. We wouldn't make it to the playoffs that year, but we did make life miserable for a bunch of other teams trying to get there.

Somehow I made it through the 1978 season without missing a game. While things were looking up for the Chargers, my future was increasingly uncertain.

One Sick Puppy

Once the season was over, I knew I had to find a way to try to stabilize my inflammatory bowel disease. I couldn't go through another season like I had just gone through, and I didn't want to even consider the possibility of surgery. Remember, professional football is a ruthless business where the weak and the sick are discarded. Besides, everyone felt that the Chargers would be in the playoff hunt, and I wanted to be part of the chase.

Meanwhile, I was still experiencing piercing cramps, bouts of nausea, and nonstop diarrhea. I spent the entire six-month off-season reading everything I could find, learning as much as I could, and trying every treatment imaginable to get rid of the disease.

In order to keep my weight up, the team trainers and a nutritionist came up with a plan to supplement my diet with special high-caloric "milkshakes" brimming with amino acids and carbohydrates. The problem was that I had to drink fifteen of those vile purple-colored concoctions each day. They tasted so bad that I had to literally plug my nose in order to get them down. It was no fun, but I would do almost anything to keep kicking.

When the 1979 season opened, I had regained some of my weight and appeared to be relatively stable. At least, that is what I tried to convince myself was happening. The season started with a bang as I kicked four field goals in our opening game win over the Seattle Seahawks. We were off and running, but with each game, I realized that it was just a matter of time. Following every kick, the pain was so excruciating that I had to sit down on the bench and wait out the piercing abdominal cramps knifing through my gut.

Several weeks later, we traveled to Boston to play the New England Patriots. In pre-game warm-ups, I could barely kick a 35-yarder with a stiff wind at my back. It was clear that my prolonged battle with IBD was taking its toll. How long could I hold out? How long before I would cost the team with my inability to kick a long-range field goal?

Those thoughts haunted me as I boarded the team plane following our disappointing loss to the Patriots. I was not looking forward to the long, cross-country flight home.

Not long after take-off, I began to feel feverish while intense cramps assaulted me. My world started spinning, and I must have blacked out. When I came to I was on fire—103 degrees! Despite my high temperature, my body shivered with chills. Someone alerted the team doctor, who quickly ordered my teammates to carefully lay me across three seats and wrap me in several blankets. They applied ice packs to my forehead as I shook violently with the fever that ravaged my insides.

The team doctor knew I was very sick and felt I would have to be hospitalized upon touchdown in San Diego. When we finally landed, however, I was feeling somewhat better, and I convinced my parents to take me to their house rather than to the hospital. In my mind, I still wasn't willing to give in and admit I couldn't go on any more.

Two days later, a panel of my doctors made the decision for me, however, and I was admitted to University Hospital in San Diego. My season was over just four games after it had begun, but more importantly, the inevitable had finally come to pass . . . I would need surgery. One year of debilitating diarrhea and stomach cramps had taken its toll. I was worn out. I had tried everything I knew to try, but I just couldn't fight it anymore. The disease was not in my head, as so many uninformed people had suggested, but was a real physical ailment that not only was threatening my career but also my life.

Dr. Gerald Peskin, my surgeon, explained that he would most likely perform a resection, or the removal of the diseased part of my bowel. He didn't believe I would need an ostomy, one of my deepest fears, but he had me sign consent papers nonetheless. The problem was that since I was so weak from my extended battle with the disease, he felt it would be necessary to wait two weeks while TPN feedings built up my strength.

I was feeling pretty sorry for myself as I lay in the hospital room watching my football career vanish right before my eyes. This is not fair. This shouldn't be happening to me. Not now . . . not when the team is just getting good and my kicking career is taking off.

Just then one of my attending physicians came in. Dr. Cammy Mowery had impressed me with her sensitivity when we had first been introduced. Now, the pent-up fears and uncertainties came tumbling out. "Is this ever going to end?" I whined. "Am I ever going to get over this?" I was so miserable that I was sobbing.

Dr. Mowery listened quietly and seemed to understand my desperation. "You want to know the truth, Rolf? The truth is you're not the first to go through this. We have a half-dozen other people on the floor with inflammatory bowel disease right now. And across the nation, there are hundreds—make that thousands—of other people in hospitals with exactly the same thing you have. The point is your situation is not unique. I know a little bit about your background in football, and I have great confidence that you can get through this." She squeezed my hand as she comforted me.

Meanwhile, abdominal cramps continued to leave me in great distress, particularly after the now-routine instances of explosive diarrhea. A blood work-up revealed that I was getting toxic and indicated the presence of bacteria in my bloodstream. My doctors decided surgery could not wait, so they scheduled the operation for the following morning.

It was quite by chance, or maybe it wasn't, that Dr. Larry Saidman, the anesthesiologist, stopped by that afternoon to check up on me and see whether I had any questions. He found me passed out in the bathroom.

When I came to, sweat was beading up on my forehead and running in rivulets down the sides of my face. My hands trembled, and I had trouble focusing on his words. My body, which was experiencing severe septic shock, shook violently from the fever.

Realizing the gravity of my situation, Dr. Saidman immediately called Dr. Peskin while I was prepped before being rushed into the operating room. After some discussion, the decision was made to proceed with the resection. A twelve-inch long incision was made on my abdomen, and my ascending colon and part of my transverse colon were snipped out. The doctors then reconnected the end of my small intestine to the remaining transverse colon and stitched me back together.

I had dodged the ostomy bullet, but had no idea that my real medical problems were just beginning.

Fevers and Spikes

After any major abdominal surgery, it's critical to keep expanding the lungs to lessen the possibility of developing pneumonia. That's why I was connected to a respirator in the Intensive Care Unit, which forced me to take deep breaths.

With each heave, however, my lacerated stomach muscles screamed in pain. Shortly after arriving in the ICU, I began experiencing fever spikes. Out of nowhere, my temperature would shoot up, but my teeth would begin chattering violently while my body shook uncontrollably. It felt as though my incision was being ripped open with each shake. These episodes lasted for up to forty-five minutes, and I would lie helplessly shaking, shivering with cold on the outside, but burning up inside.

Those horrible chills and fever spikes tormented me for days. My temperature would often get up to 104 or 105 degrees—dangerously high. Only doses of morphine eased the pain; ice packs, Tylenol, and a water mattress helped control the fevers. I was a very sick young man who was fast losing hope.

The mystery behind the unexplained fevers was revealed when cultures indicated the presence of gram-negative organisms—E. coli bacteria in my blood. My doctors feared I had either an abscess or a leak in the suture line where the two ends of my intestine had been sewn together—a critical complication that causes people to die.

"Dr. Peskin, what's going on?" I pleaded as he stopped by on one of his twice-daily visits.

"Well, we're not exactly sure," he replied, looking at my chart. "But it appears we can't wait any longer. I'm afraid that we're going to have to go back in and find out."

"You mean another surgery?" I looked at him through horrified eyes. "Are you talking about cutting me up again?"

"Rolf, there's something clearly wrong. We have no choice," Dr. Peskin answered gravely. "We have to find out what went wrong and fix it."

Six days after my initial resection, Dr. Peskin and his team sliced me open again and peered into my abdominal cavity for a second time. They quickly found the problem. A small leak at the suture line where the ileum and the colon had been reconnected had become a big gaping hole. The bacteria that normally live in my gut were now spilling into my abdomen and getting into my bloodstream, causing acute peritonitis.

"My God, look at that infection!" Dr. Peskin exclaimed to the other doctors. "I hope we caught it in time. Any longer, and the Chargers would definitely be looking for a new kicker."

The inevitable happened next—an ostomy . . . actually two ostomies. The doctors carefully snipped another inch off the end of my ileum, than began plotting where to locate the functioning ileostomy on the right side of my torso. This was where an appliance would now collect my fecal waste.

But because my surgery had been performed under emergency conditions, and because I was so sick, my doctors didn't believe I would have survived the time it would take to do a total colectomy, where my entire colon and rectum would be removed. Because of this, they were forced to create a second stoma to secure the remaining part of my colon. Rather than just leaving the rest of my large intestine to flop around inside my abdomen, they created a mucous fistula colostomy that would hold my non-functioning colon in place. It would require a bag to collect the epithelial cells that slough off the lining of the colon, but otherwise served no other purpose.

Normally, ostomy surgeries are well planned, and careful attention is paid to where the stomas are placed on the body. Stomas are generally located below the belt line so that the appliances are out of the way and the patient's belt does not restrict the opening.

For reasons I cannot fathom to this day, my stoma was mistakenly placed above my belt line. Perhaps the doctors weren't paying close attention because my surgery was performed under such stressful conditions, or perhaps the doctors just miscalculated. At any rate, stomas located above the belt line make for difficult lifestyle complications later.

To close me up, doctors sewed large wire sutures into the incision that started under my sternum and traveled south past my belly button to just above my pubic bone. Now that I was an ostomate, the NFL seemed like a world away.

Struggling Each Day

I was in bad shape when the nurses wheeled me back from the Recovery Room to the ICU. When I groggily came to and learned that an ostomy had been performed, I couldn't believe it. I was numb. Surely when I went back to sleep and woke up I would learn that this was all just some kind of bad dream. Did they really say I had two bags?

During the few lucid moments between my drug-induced naps, I wondered whether life was really worth fighting for. What was the point? I would never be able to kick in the NFL again. Worse, I would never again participate in the other sports and outdoor activities I loved. From where I was lying, my life was all but over. When the nurses changed my dressings for the first time and I caught a glimpse of my horribly cut-up stomach, I received visual confirmation that things were bad . . . really bad.

As if to make matters worse, I was seized again by shaking chills. For days the fevers raged, and my resting pulse more than doubled. I felt ice cold and begged for warm blankets. Each day was a monumental struggle. I didn't realize it at the time, but I was in a real battle for my life.

Four days after my surgery, Melba Conner, an enterostomal therapy nurse, gave me my first ileostomy lesson. Barely coherent at the time, I wasn't much in the mood to deal with my ostomy. There was too much else going on to come to grips with the fact that I would have to live with a bag.

Melba was persistent, however, and when I found out she had an ileostomy of her own, I grudgingly listened. It turned out that she had loads of experience and had actually become one of the first ET nurses in the country. She talked openly about living with an appliance, what I could expect, and how little it would change my lifestyle. Still, I was overwhelmed at everything happening to me.

"I don't know, Melba. I'm not sure I can handle all of this," I said, barely choking back tears.

"It's not a question of whether you can handle it," she stated firmly. "There is simply no option. Besides, if it weren't for the surgery, you'd be six feet under right now. Remember that always."

I stared at her. She had my attention now.

"I know this is an enormous change for anybody," she continued, "and maybe more so for someone as athletic as you. Listen, I don't follow football much, but I've never heard the nurses talk about a patient getting so much mail. You must have a lot of friends out there who care about you, so if I were you, I'd start by being thankful for my blessings."

I nodded and continued to listen.

"Now, let's get to the basics," said Melba, as she touched my stoma with her index finger. "It's going to seem like a lot of information at first, but for now, just watch what I do."

I shook my head and closed my eyes. *If only those bags would disappear.*

"Look, Rolf," she said, as if she was reading my mind. "These appliances are not going away. You have to learn how they work. For the rest of your life, you're going to have to do this. If you learn well, they shouldn't interfere with anything you do—anything!"

Melba took my hand and had me touch my left stoma. It was shiny, a bit wet-looking, and dark pink—not unlike the lining of my mouth. The one-inch round stoma protruded from my left side about half an inch.

Melba explained that there weren't any nerve endings in the stoma, so touching couldn't hurt. The stoma's redness meant it was well vascularized, she continued, adding that I may notice a little blood—perfectly natural and no cause for alarm—when changing the appliance.

"You're lucky to have had your surgery now and not ten years ago," she said. "Modern appliances today allow you to go five or six days before changing faceplates. They are easy on your skin, won't leak or smell, and no one has to know you are wearing one. It wasn't so long ago that virtually nothing was available. Patients would have to create their own "bag," using old rubber heating water bottles, cans, plastic bags, or whatever else they could come up with. They would leak and smell, and the corrosion on a person's skin was absolutely horrendous."

"Maybe I am fortunate," I said with a little optimism, and the first positive thought I'd had in a while.

"You are," she replied. "Now let's change those appliances of yours."

Melba gently removed my old appliances and cleaned around the stomas with soap and water. She was careful not to snag anything on my protruding wire sutures or touch my painful incision. Then she dried around them with a towel and used a skin prep to clean the area. Next, she cut two stoma-sized holes out of a pair of faceplate barriers that would snugly sit around the stomas to protect my skin from the burning digestive enzymes. Before she attached them, however, she spread a whitish paste around my stomas and waited several minutes for the glue to get tacky. (Paste is not necessary with nearly all of today's appliances.)

With the gentleness of someone who had done this a thousand times before, she carefully fitted the faceplates over my stomas one at a time and pressed firmly to seal them. After adding some paper tape around the faceplate borders, she attached the new pouches, which snapped into a secure position. *Voila!* I had new appliances. The whole process took only ten minutes and seemed relatively simple.

Melba checked the clip on the bag collecting the

waste. "When you're up and around, you're going to need to empty your pouch six or seven times a day," she explained. "It will depend on how much you eat and drink. You'll learn very quickly how your digestive system works and how fast your bag fills up."

"How am I going to empty it?" I asked, still trying to take it all in.

"When you sit on the toilet; position the bag between your legs, release the clip, and the contents of the bag will drain into the bowl. When you're done, take some tissue and clean the end of the bag, fold it and fasten the clip, and you're on your way."

"Okay," I replied skeptically, "but what about the smell?"

"Not a problem. The new appliances today are so good they prevent that. The only odor you will have is when you empty the pouch in the bathroom. But, that's no different from any normal person."

Melba smiled, seeming to know just what I was thinking. "Don't worry, you're going to do just fine. There may even be a day when you will actually look back at all of this and count your blessings. Life has a funny way of getting our attention and then making sure we learn what is really important."

Making a Comeback

I'm not going to sugarcoat what happened over the next month in the hospital. Complications set in, and I almost needed a third surgery. I was exhausted and depressed. I hated the constant blood draws, the changing of my IVs and dressings, and the many ways I lost my dignity. The morphine and other painkillers caused hallucinations and made sleep difficult.

But I also experienced God's mercy and the love of my family and friends. I learned to live moment-by-moment and what it took to get through each day. I tried not to worry about the future and, instead, focused on my little "victories." It was a milestone when I could get out of bed without assistance, walk three trips down the hall instead of two, and blow my breathing apparatus and finally make the ball go all the way to the top five times in a row.

When it came time to be discharged, my doctors decided that I should spend the first few weeks recuperating at my parent's house. Upon arrival, I weighed myself on the family scale. I was down to one hundred and twenty-six pounds, almost sixty pounds below what I was listed at in the Chargers' media guide!

I turned to my mother and smirked, "My new playing weight."

What wasn't so amusing was learning to change my appliances for the first time without Melba's help. The prospect frightened me.

The day finally came. Mom and I carefully arranged all of the supplies in front of us and began the procedure by cutting the faceplates. No sooner had we removed one of the worn-out appliances when the stoma began to ooze. Caught unprepared, all we could do was watch in horror as the waste matter leaked onto my stomach and slid slowly onto my clothes. Of course, the foul smell was not pleasant for either of us.

We quickly wiped up and continued.

"We've got to clean the skin around the stoma before we apply the adhesive paste," Mom reminded me.

Sensing some urgency, Mom began to help me with the skin prep, but as if on cue, the stoma began to ooze again. In the fumbling for a towel, Mom managed to drop the paste container on the floor and knock over a glass of water next to me on the table.

"Not again!" Mom said in a frustrated voice.

We were living Murphy's Law: Anything that could go wrong did go wrong. We made four or five attempts at cleaning around the stoma, prepping the skin, and applying the paste before we were finally able to position the stupid bag. A procedure that should have taken no longer than the time it takes to kick a game-winning field goal took us forty-five agonizing minutes.

"This is ridiculous," I declared in anger. "Is the rest of my life going to be like this?"

It would take several more stabs at changing my appliances to get the hang of them, weeks to get back on my feet, and months to heal. As I slowly began to regain my strength and learn to live with the appliances, I began to wonder secretly if I could possibly kick again. Without telling anyone except the Charger's conditioning coach, I became a man on a mission and set my sights on the opening of training camp in July.

If I successfully regained my position on the team, I would become the first NFL player to compete while wearing an ostomy appliance, but that prospect seemed like light years away. First, I had to convince the doctors and myself that I could properly protect the stomas and convince the skeptics that I could kick again.

I don't think my coaches held out much hope when training camp finally rolled around that summer, but I had worked very hard to get back into shape and kicked well. What finally sealed the deal and won my job back was kicking a 55-yarder in our third preseason game.

I ended up playing seven more seasons in the NFL, experiencing some great moments along the way. I was named Comeback Player of the Year in 1980, earned a spot in the Pro Bowl in 1982, and was named the NFL "Man of the Year" in 1983. My career highlight was kicking the game-winning field goal against the Miami Dolphins in a 1982 playoff game that *Sports Illustrated* would later call the second greatest game in NFL history.

My football career was a lot of fun, but when I got sick with ulcerative colitis, I was forced to learn that there was more to life than Sunday afternoon football games. I learned that while life is not always fair, we have a choice: we can fold out of the game, or we can play the hand we have been dealt and hope that the next hand is better. I feel so fortunate that so many people encouraged me to keep at it, people who convinced me that life is always worth fighting for, no matter how difficult it may seem at the time.

I am now married to an incredible wife, Mary, and we have four very special children. Our lives are rich beyond measure, and I realize now that God has gifted me with a second chance at life, just like the individuals you'll meet in the stories that follow. I hope these people inspire you—or a family member—to not only survive whatever you are going through, but to thrive.

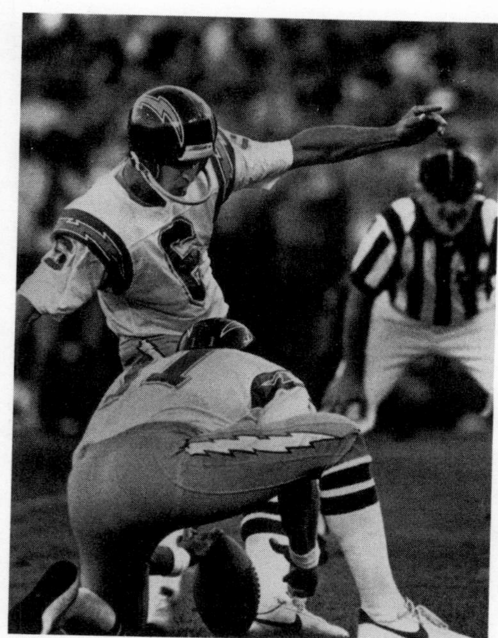

I went from kicking field goals for the San Diego Chargers on Sundays to wondering if life was worth living following my ostomy surgery in 1979. Wire sutures held my surgical incision together (below).

Once I resumed my NFL kicking career, I started "Kicks for Critters," a program to educate and raise funds for the preservation of endangered species through the San Diego Zoo (bottom left). We were able to raise $2 million dollars.

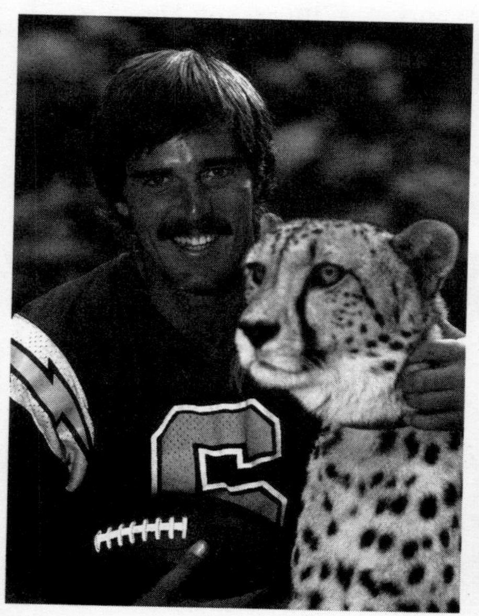

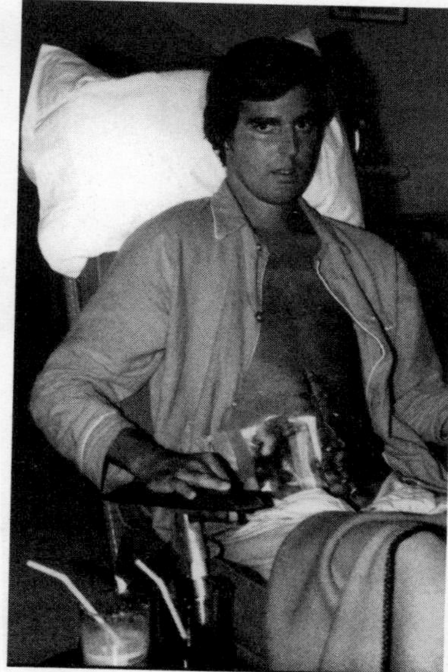

One of the benefits of surviving ostomy surgery has been the opportunity to encourage others. I accompanied Irene Fine, a remarkable ostomy patient from Russia, on a visit to the Oval Office to meet President George Bush in 1990.

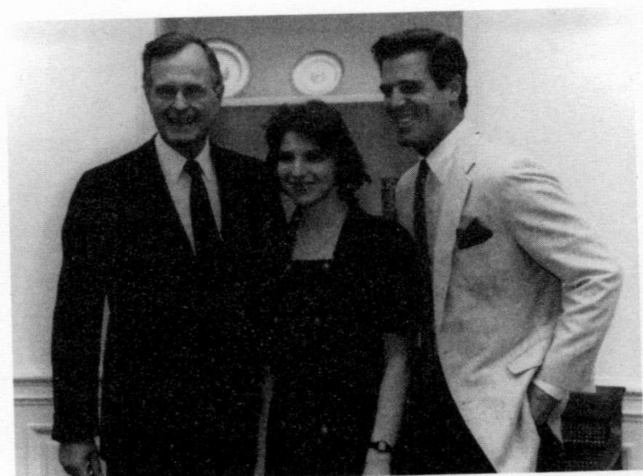

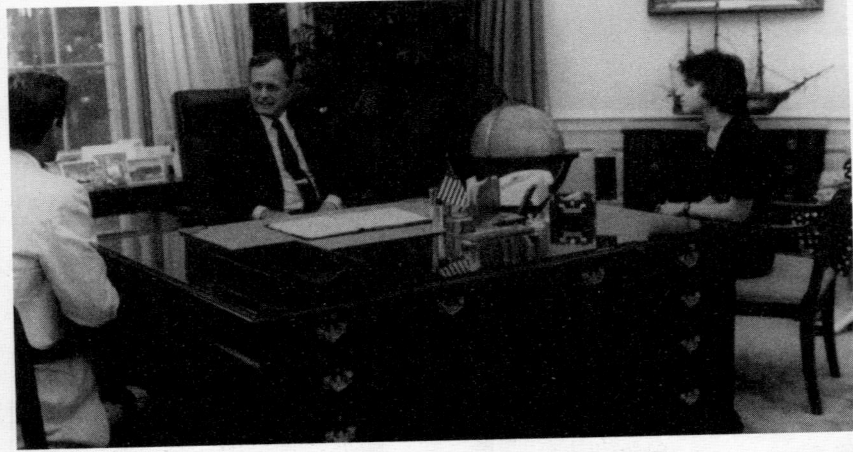

I also had the chance to meet former White House press secretary James Brady, who survived a serious gunshot wound during the assassination attempt on President Reagan in 1981.

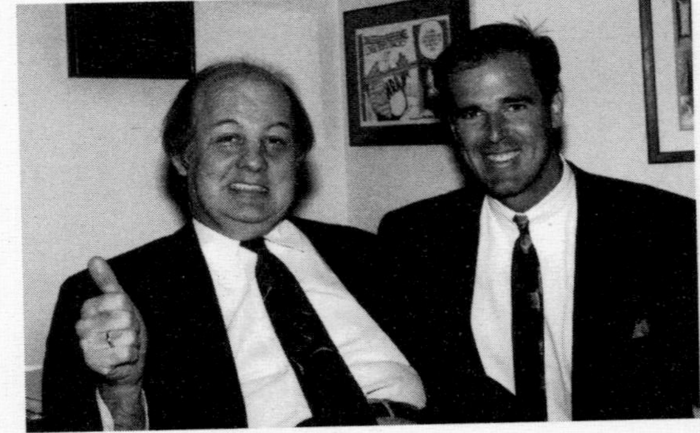

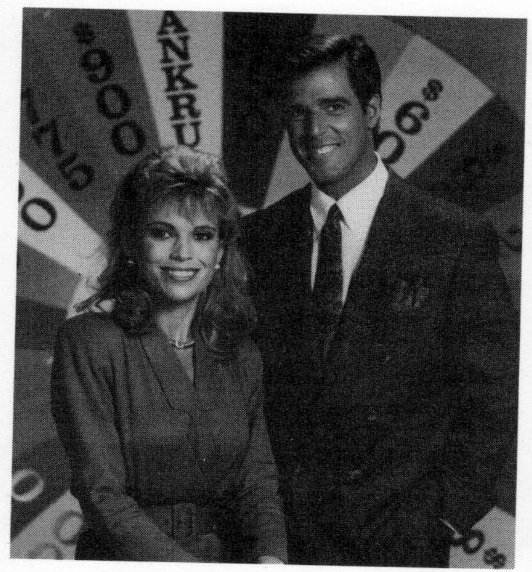

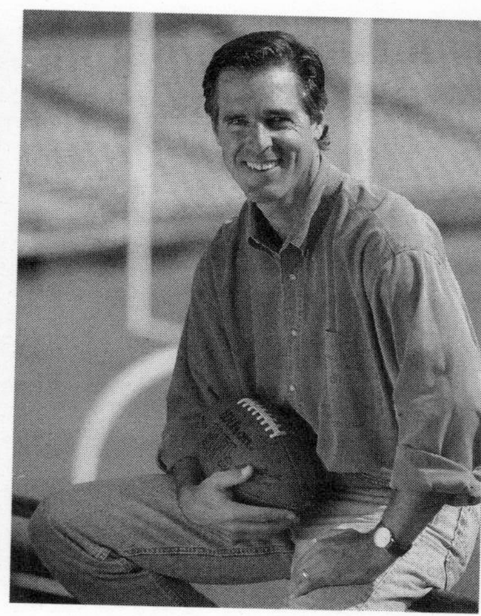

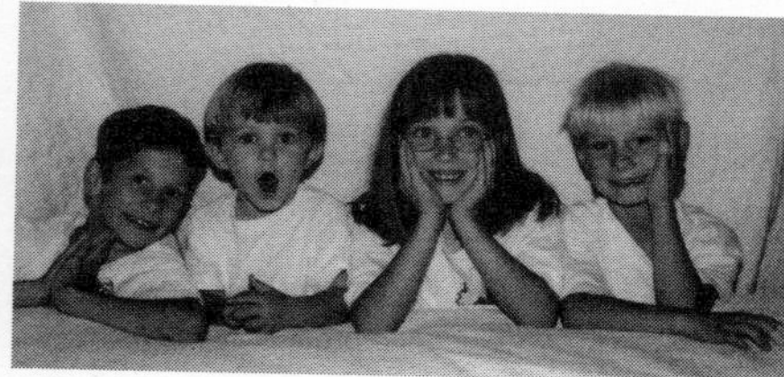

Yes, I enjoyed my fifteen minutes of fame during my one-season stint in 1989 as the host of the "Wheel of Fortune" game show with Vanna White. What's most important in my life is my family: my wife, Mary, and our four children, Kari, Erik, Ryan, and Timmy (bottom photo).

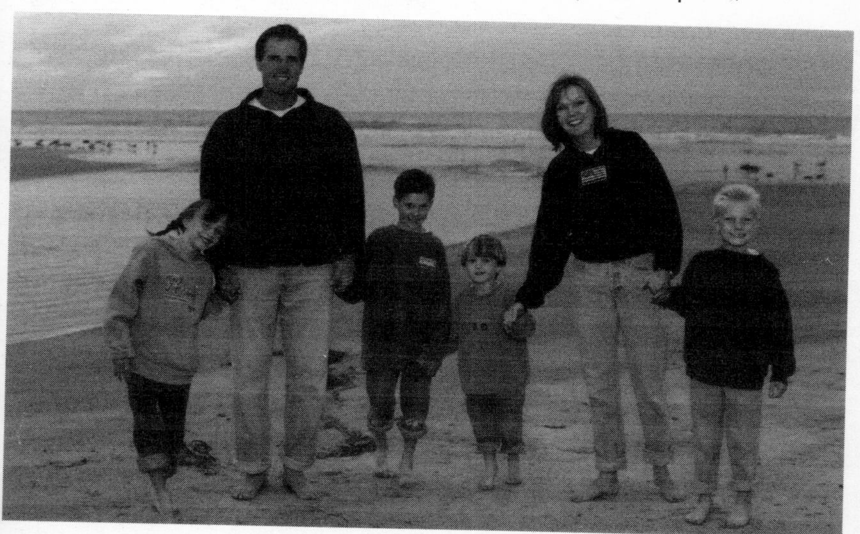

One Day at a Time

VALENCIA HARDAWAY

AGE

31

HOMETOWN

Atlanta, Georgia

MEDICAL SITUATION

After a difficult battle with ulcerative colitis that almost ended her life, Valencia underwent ileostomy surgery at the age of twenty-four.

Valencia Hardaway cracks two eggs into a bowl, adds a splash of milk, and begins whipping the eggs with a fork. She pours the mixture into a hot pan sizzling with margarine, reaches for the toaster to drop in a slice of bread, and then gently scrambles the eggs.

When the eggs are done, she sets the steaming plate, along with a plastic cup of juice and a slice of toast, jellied and quartered, on the table before a four-year-old boy named Stephon. The child smiles and thanks his aunt before plunging his Winnie-the-Pooh fork into his breakfast.

"The eggs are hot," Valencia warns, tucking a napkin into the little boy's pajama top. "Blow on them first." She returns the smile before going back to the sink to clean up.

Such ordinary things—cooking breakfast for her sister's son, standing on her own two feet in the kitchen, or opening her mouth to speak. There was a time when even these simple tasks seemed improbable for Valencia Hardaway.

The Early Days

Valencia was one of those kids who never got sick. All through school she was vibrant and healthy, never even catching the ubiquitous childhood chicken pox. If anything, Valencia's biggest battle was with her weight, though this never prevented her from making the cheerleading squad in junior high and all through high school. A devout Christian, Valencia used to pray that God would take the extra pounds away from her. Little did she know that the weight would come off, but not in the way she expected.

In 1988, after graduating in the Top Ten of her high school class, Valencia opted for the career path of cosmetology rather than a four-year college. In 1991 she earned her Master Cosmetologist license and honed her craft for two years at Xavier's Hair Design in her hometown of Atlanta before deciding to head out on her own.

In 1993, she and her mother's sister, Dorothy, opened their own hair salon. They called it "D and V's"—Dorothy and Valencia's. Though the two women started from scratch—two chairs in a corner of a shared office building—they had big dreams. They were going to make something out of this place. Overseeing the installation of new sinks and floors, they transformed their corner of the office on a shoestring budget. Their do-it-yourself decorating included wallpaper and curtains, pictures and house plants. When the salon opened, it quickly earned a reputation for quality service. Gradually, their clientele grew.

Meanwhile, Valencia found an apartment—a nice, one-bedroom unit in nearby Decatur, and she even bought herself a new car. At twenty-three, she was independent financially and emotionally, with a stable future in a career she loved. Life couldn't get much better than this.

And then she got sick.

It began one afternoon while doing a bob on a new client. Valencia loved the challenge of taking an unfamiliar head of hair and creating an entirely new look. The cut was going well; the client seemed relaxed and satisfied. Earlier that day, Valencia had splurged and eaten a cheeseburger for lunch—something she hadn't done for a while as she was still trying to lose a few pounds. Halfway through the haircut, her stomach began to cramp. Rather than push through the appointment and risk ruining the cut, she excused herself to use the restroom, where she had a violent episode of diarrhea.

She returned to her client and managed to finish the day at work before dragging herself home. Assuming she'd had an adverse reaction to the greasy fries from lunch, she swore off junk food and went to bed early, hoping she'd feel better in the morning.

She did feel better—until she swallowed some toast and juice for breakfast. Within minutes, she was in the bathroom, experiencing another bout of cramping and diarrhea. She called her aunt, told her she was sick, and asked her to cancel her appointments. "Maybe I can try to double up some clients during the evenings next week," she suggested. "I'm sure I'll be better by tomorrow."

Valencia hung up the phone, frustrated and annoyed. She really couldn't afford to miss a day of work. She made a cup of tea, put a few crackers on a plate and went to the couch to try and get some rest. She sipped on her tea and nibbled on a cracker. Within minutes, she was rushing to the bathroom.

A Rising Concern

Rosa Hardaway, Valencia's mother, was flat-out tired. She had worked overtime again at her job as senior accountant at Georgia Institute of Technology, and she was exhausted. A hot bath would be great, she thought, as she turned the key in the front door and let herself in.

There was a note on the counter from Rosa's youngest daughter, Melissa, saying she'd be home late from cheer practice. And there were two messages on the answering machine. Rosa pressed "play" and listened to them while scanning the contents of the refrigerator, trying to piece together a simple dinner. She was hungry.

Both messages were from her daughter, Valencia. She was still having trouble with her stomach and had gone to the doctor again that afternoon. He had prescribed more medication, Valencia said, this time for hemorrhoids. The last batch didn't seem to help.

That was the first message. Valencia's second message was more concise, her voice agitated and tense. *Can I stay at your place over the weekend?*

Rosa knew that this would be the third weekend in a row that her second eldest daughter "Lynn" had asked to come home and stay. Valencia was starting to spend more time at Mom's home than at her apartment, mainly because she was so sick. Mom, naturally, was concerned why her daughter's appetite had decreased so much.

No matter how much tender loving care she received on the weekends, Lynn didn't seem to be getting any better. *How long will it be,* Rosa thought, *before these doctors figure out what's wrong with my daughter?* All these pills don't seem to do a thing. If anything, Lynn seems to be getting worse. And she has to endure those horrible rectal exams each time she visits the doctor. Would it never end?

> *I had never been sick before, so I didn't know what to expect.*
>
> *I believed the doctors were doing whatever they could to help me.*
>
> *You just figure they know what they're doing . . .*

Two months after signing a one-year lease on her apartment, Valencia Hardaway moved back into her mother's house. She was so ill that she could no longer work and was forced to leave the salon in her Aunt Dorothy's care. The burden to sustain the business was too much, however, and they eventually lost the salon.

Valencia hardly noticed. She went from bedroom to toilet every thirty minutes, passing so much blood rectally she would sometimes collapse on the floor of the bathroom. She began sleeping by a portable heater just to keep warm. And she slept. In between bathroom visits, it seemed all she did was sleep.

Rosa was becoming desperate. Each week, she would take Valencia to the doctor. Each week, a different doctor would probe and prod, and then he would prescribe another medication. It was, Valencia would say later, as if they had no idea what to do with her and were merely guessing. Oddly enough, the doctors never checked her blood.

One afternoon, Rosa noticed that her daughter seemed more lethargic than usual. And her lips seemed so pale. Something seemed to connect in her mind, something about blood loss and anemia. But wouldn't those doctors have checked for this? On impulse, Rosa called her primary care physician and made an appointment for her daughter. She dragged Valencia out of bed and literally carried her to the car and into the doctor's office.

Once there, the nurse did a finger prick in order to get a reading, but she couldn't draw any blood. She tried again and again. Concerned that something was wrong with the machine, the nurse informed the doctor of the problem. He took one look at Valencia and needed no one to tell him that the machine wasn't broken. He picked up the phone and arranged for Valencia to be transported to DeKalb Medical Hospital. Later he told Rosa that if Valencia had slept another day, she would most likely have slipped into a coma.

At Dekalb, Valencia received ten pints of blood. She was also examined by a gastroenterologist, who for the first time diagnosed Valencia with ulcerative colitis. He informed her that her colon was so diseased that the only option left was to have it surgically removed. Had he seen her earlier, perhaps he could have done something for her.

> *They said I'd only have to wear the pouch for about six weeks, and then they'd reverse it.*
>
> *That's what kept me going. I could never live with a pouch for the rest of my life.*
>
> *Never.*

On March 16, 1994, Valencia went into the operating room for ileostomy surgery. She awoke to intense pain and an ostomy pouch on her side. Reminding herself that the pouch was only temporary, she set her sights on the day she would be well enough to have the procedure reversed.

But Valencia didn't get well. Two months later, she had a second operation, this time to deal with a fistula. From then on, from Easter to Christmas and every holiday in between, she was back in for more surgery. Each time, the same incision would be re-opened, from sternum to pelvis. Each time, Valencia would wait for the inevitable chills that would set her limbs shivering and remind her once again that she couldn't go home, not yet.

A growing sense that she would never get well came over her like the summer heat that suffocates Atlanta. The hope that had kept her going—that the ileostomy would be reversed—gradually faded. Valencia began to despair. She was tired. Tired of hospitals. Tired of pain. Tired of the wretched ostomy pouch. Indeed, she would have nothing to do with it; she wouldn't even touch it. She turned her face away when her mother changed it for her. She hated the sounds of the hospital and the stench of her own excrement. She despised her life. She was ready to die. No, more than that. She wanted to die.

A Tough Go

It was Christmas, that same year. Valencia had been home long enough to see the pretty lights on the tree before returning, once again, to the hospital for yet another surgery—her seventh. That morning her mother called, as she always did, to check on her daughter and to let her know what time she'd be coming in.

Rosa, who finally had to quit her job in order to care for Valencia full time, listened as her daughter spoke, then asked, "Valencia, have you been exerting yourself?"

She hadn't.

"Then why are you breathing so hard?"

Valencia hadn't noticed.

That was a Saturday morning. Rosa's youngest daughter was still asleep and the house was quiet. After telling Valencia she'd be there later that day, she hung up the phone.

Less than an hour later, at 9:00 a.m., the phone rang. It was St. Joseph's Hospital. Valencia had been transferred to the ICU and was being prepped for emergency surgery. Her heart rate was skyrocketing, and her fever had spiked. Rosa found out later that in addition to a bowel obstruction, pelvic sepsis, and liver lacerations, the infection had spread to Valencia's lungs.

Somehow Rosa managed to make the hour-long drive to the hospital and arrive, breathless and panting, in time to see her daughter being wheeled out of ICU, on her way to surgery. When Valencia, who'd had to sign her own consent form for the surgery, saw her mother, she began crying uncontrollably, and then gasping for air. Immediately an oxygen mask was placed over her face causing Valencia to panic and grab for the mask. It was the last thing she remembers.

> *People ask me if I saw God.*
>
> *I say no. But I did see a woman.*
>
> *A white woman, with long, flowing blonde hair. Which is odd, because I didn't know anyone who fit that description.*

Her fever hovered between 102 and 105 the entire time she was on life support. Twice she returned to the surgery bay during those two months, once for a tracheotomy. Valencia's lungs had turned white; massive doses of antibiotics being pumped into her body did nothing to halt the infection. The Center for Disease Control, suspecting AIDS, tested her for HIV. When the test came back negative, they shrugged their shoulders. There was nothing more to be done. Taking her off life support was the only thing left to do.

By this time, Rosa had moved into the hospital, camping out in the waiting room, sleeping on two chairs pushed together, and brushing her teeth in the ladies' room. Christmas came and went and Rosa was still there, keeping vigil; talking to her daughter; caressing her arms and legs; praying . . . always praying. The doctors gave Rosa the weekend to decide her course of action: either allow them to open Valencia up again to look at her lungs or remove her from life support altogether.

Rosa was adamant. Valencia had been cut upon enough. No more surgery. The doctors had done everything humanly possible to save Valencia's life. They had tried everything and had even covered the Hardaways' astronomical medical bills. Now it was in God's hands. She went home and prayed: *If you're going to take her, go ahead and do it. But I can't make the decision to take her off life support.*

The phone rang the following Monday morning. It was the hospital. Valencia's fever had just broken. It was a few days after the New Year.

I couldn't tell them that what they were doing hurt me. When I hurt, I held up a card that said PAIN. That was how they knew.

Valencia's recovery was slow, painful and grueling. There was the agony of withdrawal from the drugs that had been coursing through her body; the failed attempts to speak that sent her into violent coughing spasms; the physical therapy, where all she could do at first was sit up for twenty-minute sessions.

As difficult as recovery was, though, something had changed. Hope had replaced despair. As though someone had tossed her a life raft, Valencia knew it was now up to her to grab hold and climb in. She'd been given a second chance. If that second chance included accepting the ostomy pouch for the rest of her life, then so be it. Who was she to complain? Then again, there was still that tiny, flickering hope. Maybe some day. . . .

The Road Back

Valencia Hardaway went home from the hospital in January 1995 with the will to live. Five months later in June, she returned to the hospital, this time to close the ileostomy. A month later, however, she was back, with an infection. She spent three days getting her stomach pumped of mucous and pus. She returned the following month for a fistulotomy.

It was no use. Every time Valencia's doctor tried to reverse the ostomy, infection would set in. The time had come, her doctor said, to choose between chronic illness and infection, or living a productive life. Valencia had no other choice. Her final surgery took place that August. When she awoke, it was to the stark reality that this time there was no turning back. The ostomy would be permanent. Like waking up after surgery for the first time, she was devastated.

It was during this last hospital stay that Valencia's attitude about her whole ordeal would change. While shuffling down the hospital corridors following her surgery, Valencia happened to glance into a room where she saw a young white woman, not quite twenty, lying in a bed. She had long, beautiful blond hair. Something about her prompted Valencia to step into the room.

Her name was Shannan. Like Valencia, she, too, had ulcerative colitis and was scheduled to have ostomy surgery. And like Valencia, she was devastated. She would rather die than go through life with a bag, she told Valencia.

How well Valencia knew! Even now, after having been given this second chance at life, Valencia understood. But she couldn't say so. She had to be strong—for someone else. Instead, she held her hand as the girl cried herself to sleep. During her next visit, she promised Shannan that she would be with her when it was time for her to go into surgery. And she kept that promise. She was with her then; was with her for successive surgeries; and, two years later, she was with her again—on Shannan's wedding day and the subsequent birth of her son, Skyler.

Perhaps it was then—as she watched the girl who had all but given up on life, exchange wedding vows with her husband-to-be—that Valencia recalled the vision of a blond-haired girl when her own life hung by a thread. Was Shannon the same girl in her vision? And why the vision? Was her life spared in order to give hope to another? Was she a sign from God to help define Valencia's purpose for living?

These were thoughts worth pondering.

Meanwhile, though, her own life stretched before her. There were things to do. People to help. Dreams to pursue.

And a little boy to care for.

Valencia Hardaway lives with her mother in Atlanta while making plans to open a new hair salon. She continues to take care of her nephew, Stephon, while her sister attends college. Valencia has followed through with her promise, and she speaks often to encourage others facing ostomy surgery.

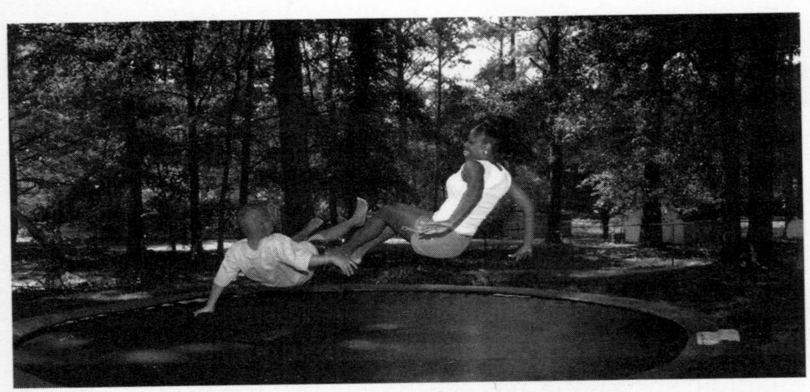

Nobody can say that Valencia Hardaway didn't bounce back from ostomy surgery. She's a devout young woman who believes God helped pull her through her most difficult days.

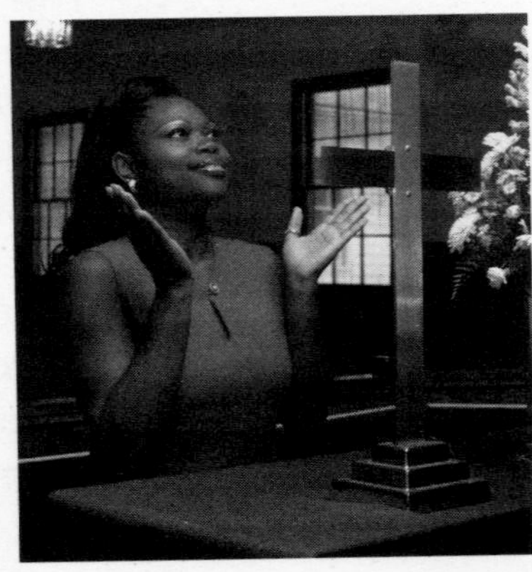

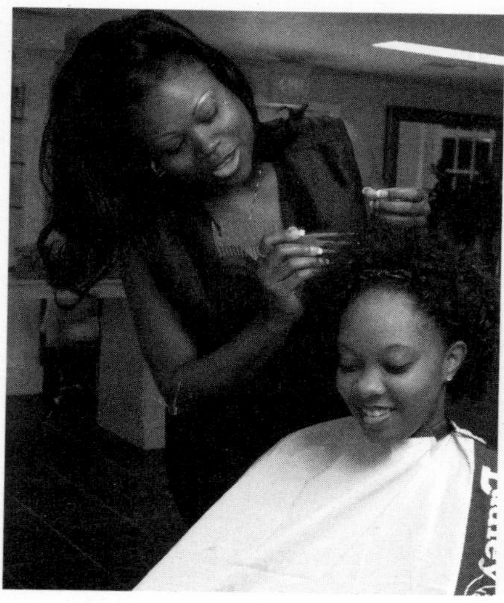

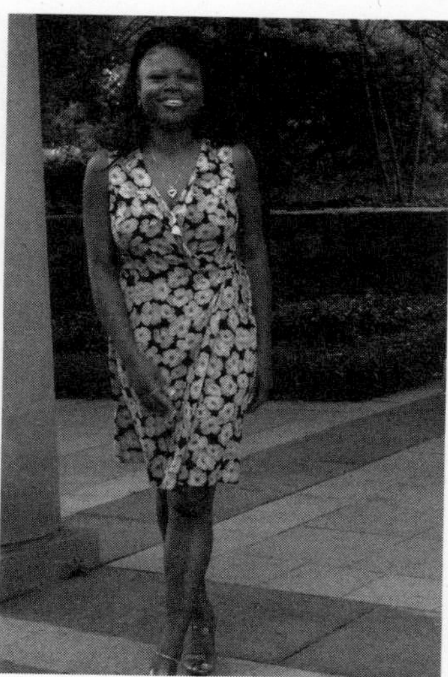

Valencia had to sell her fledgling hair salon business when she was hit full force with ulcerative colitis. These days, this confident young woman from Atlanta is planning a comeback in the hair-styling business while she helps out her sister by looking after her nephew, Stephon.

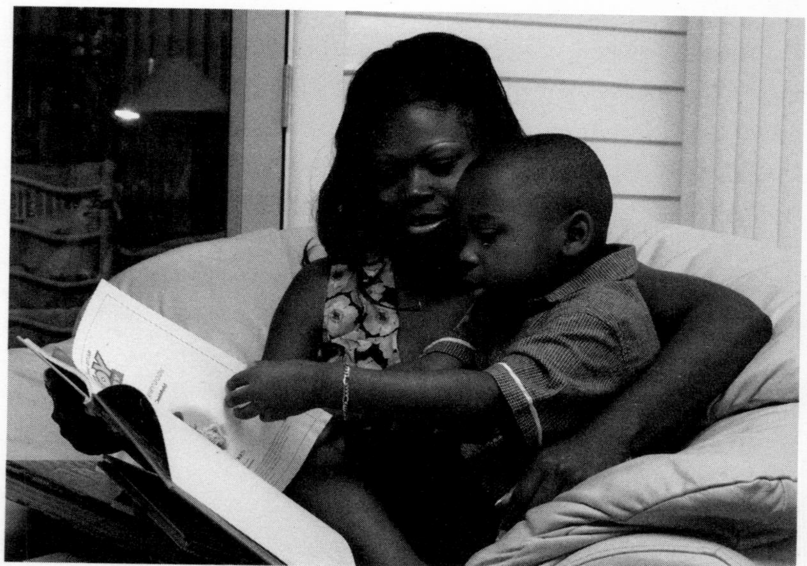

Photographs by Susanne Callan of ConvaTec, a division of Bristol Myers-Squibb.

BACK TO THE FUTURE

MARVIN BUSH

AGE
45

HOMETOWN
Alexandria, Virginia

MEDICAL SITUATION
Seemingly overnight and at the most awkward of times, he developed ulcerative colitis and needed ileostomy surgery at the age of twenty-nine.

He describes himself as a forward-looking man—which may explain why he's fuzzy on the details. He can't remember, for example, how old he was when he first started getting sick. Or how long he endured the symptoms of ulcerative colitis before he realized this could be serious business. He's even reluctant to talk about those dark days lying in a hospital bed—days long gone and sooner forgotten.

Piece together the story of Marvin Bush, and like a jigsaw puzzle missing its cover, you get a sense that this is a story both complex and beautiful. And if it seems a few pieces of the puzzle are missing, perhaps it's because the central character is a man who views the past as but a stepping stone to the future—a stone not worth turning over and examining lest the next stone be missed or overlooked.

His health began to deteriorate when he was in his late twenties. "Twenty-seven or eight—something like that," says the youngest son and fourth of six children of George and Barbara Bush. (That's George Herbert

Walker Bush, 41st President of the United States, for detail-oriented people.) In the mid-1980s—about the time his father was embarking on his second term as Vice President under Ronald Reagan—Marvin began to get sick. Married only four years to his wife, Margaret, whom he met while getting his Bachelors degree in English at the University of Virginia, he started experiencing painful cramping, bloody stools, and spiking fevers—symptoms he'd had before in varying degrees, but never all at once and never with such intensity.

Concerned, he went to see his physician. On one occasion, the doctor discovered and removed anal cysts, which made him feel better. On another, Marvin was treated for ulcers, which also seemed to alleviate the symptoms, but only briefly. What was happening, Marvin explains, is that the treatments and the medications were masking the real problem, something he suspected but didn't want to admit. Being young and active and accustomed to good health, Marvin was loath to pursue further medical guidance. He sensed that embarking on a more serious quest for an answer to his health problems would most likely lead to uncomfortable and humiliating exams at best, and at worst, the detection of serious illness.

"I thought I was bulletproof," explains the forty-five-year-old investment manager who lives with his wife and two children in northern Virginia. "I had never really been sick up until that point. And at first, the symptoms came and went. It's not as though I was ignoring the problem. I just didn't take an active enough role in trying to find a proper diagnosis."

"He had no idea of the gravity of the situation,"

adds his forty-two-year-old wife, Margaret, a former elementary school teacher and part-time actress. "It took some time for him to summon the courage to deal with the uncomfortable scopes and the tests."

The moment of reckoning came while spending a weekend with his parents in their summer home in Kennebunkport, on the southern coast of Maine, during the summer of 1985. It was the year President Ronald Reagan was diagnosed with colon cancer, and the nightly news displayed graphics of the President's digestive tract and documented his symptoms, inch by colon inch, in explicit detail.

News of President Reagan's health was more than idle curiosity for Vice President George Bush and his family, who had a vested interest in the Commander-in-Chief's health. Should President Reagan become incapacitated, or worse, should he die, the man vacationing in this idyllic oceanfront sanctuary would assume the responsibility of leading this nation. Indeed, according to Barbara Bush, for seven hours George Bush was, in fact, the president of the United States. In her published memoirs, Mrs. Bush writes that prior to Reagan's surgery, the President signed a paper transferring power to the Vice-President. The magnitude of this fact shadowed the family as they gathered in the living room and listened to the reports.

Another person in that room, however, had cause for alarm of a different nature. True, his father becoming president would make him the First Son (or one of them)—something that would give anyone pause. But as Marvin Bush listened to the doctors clicking off Reagan's symptoms one by one, he grew increasingly alarmed.

"Every symptom they listed was a symptom I had experienced. I kept nodding my head—it was like getting an A+ on a test," he says, adding that the longer he listened, the more sickened he felt, knowing that he'd put off dealing with a potentially life-threatening illness. Even Mrs. Bush seemed to make some kind of connection to what was happening on the TV screen and what little she knew about Marvin's health problems. He recalls her glancing at him periodically during the broadcast.

Until then, Marvin had not made any real effort to discuss his deteriorating health with his parents—a choice he made out of deference to them. "There was never any pressure on me not to talk about my health with my parents," he says. "At the same time, I deliberately tried not to distract them from their core responsibilities. In the final analysis, however, I am their child, and they're my mom and dad. I don't look at them as public figures."

Checking Out All Possibilities

That day in Kennebunkport, Marvin knew the time had come to deal with the issue openly. "I remember the four of us sitting in the living room," recalls Margaret. "Marvin looked at his parents and admitted that he was experiencing all of the symptoms of colon cancer. It was a moment of truth for him, in a way."

At his parents' prompting, he saw a general practitioner, Dr. Tabb Moore, whom Mrs. Bush describes in her memoirs as "an excellent doctor and a former neighbor." Rather than rush headlong into judgment, Dr. Moore decided to rule out all other possibilities before making a diagnosis. As expected, Marvin found himself undergoing humiliating and uncomfortable exams—the upper and lower GI's, the barium swallows, and the colonoscopies. It was, he says, "very, very humbling. You learn to put your dignity aside."

To his relief, cancer was eliminated early on. As a precautionary measure, however, Marvin began a drug regimen of Sulfasalzine to treat what his doctor suspected was ulcerative colitis, but the drug caused a violent allergic reaction. Marvin remembers being rushed to the hospital "looking like the Elephant Man," his skin ablaze, his face swollen and disfigured, and his throat closing up. But there was more to come.

He tried, as Mrs. Bush writes, "to go on his merry way, pretty much ignoring everything his doctor told him." Increasingly, though, the bathroom became his point of reference. He found himself needing to use the toilet at fifteen-minute intervals, a nuisance and distraction for a successful businessman and top-notch athlete, but for Marvin, it was also an indication that the situation was rapidly deteriorating. The crisis came one day while en route to California by air, with a layover in Denver. He never made it to California. Before landing in Denver, Marvin had what he calls "a bad flare-up," his way of not remembering that he was, as his wife tells it, "in excruciating pain."

Upon landing, Marvin contacted his brother who lived in the Denver area and checked himself into a local hospital before flying home as soon as he felt up for the trip. With Margaret out of town visiting family in Virginia, Marvin drove to his parents' home. There, in the Vice Presidential mansion on the grounds of the

Naval Observatory in Washington D.C., the stark reality of Marvin's condition hit his parents like ice water on a bed of coals.

"I'll never forget that day," Marvin says, in a moment of vivid recollection. "I was watching a video with Mom, but I had to go to the bathroom at least six times, causing her to hit the pause button each time. Mom is a patient person, but this was ridiculous. Then she heard me retching in the bathroom. I had lost about ten pounds by then. I was having a hard time holding food down."

Shocked by how ill he had become, Marvin's parents voiced their concern. He broke down and admitted he needed help. It was the spring of 1986. Vice President George Bush had already decided to run for President. The Bush family was in high gear, readying themselves for the challenging campaign ahead. But for Marvin, the next move was clear: Georgetown Hospital in Washington.

Test After Test

He thought it would be a brief stay. When the nurses told him to unpack his clothes and put them away in a closet, he told them it wouldn't be necessary. He figured he'd go through the tests, get the necessary drugs, and be out in the morning. He was wrong.

Marvin spent weeks in the hospital undergoing tests, with a constant procession of doctors, interns, medical students, specialists, family, and friends parading in and out of his hospital room. One of his worst moments came when an intern, who had inserted an nastogastric (NG) tube through his nose and down his throat, failed to turn up the suction high enough. Bile trickled through Marvin's nose and back down again. "Six or seven people came in on their rounds when I had vomit dribble all over my face," he recalls. "I couldn't control it. I was too tired to yell. It was one of my most degrading moments ever."

It was a few weeks later in early May 1986 when the doctors approached Marvin and tried to explain what his options were. They could either continue to try to get the disease under control using more and different drugs—the likelihood of which grew dimmer every day—or they could perform ileostomy surgery. Though he hadn't the faintest idea what they were talking about, at that point Marvin had grown so weak and was in so much pain that he was game for anything.

In retrospect, however, he believes there must have been a period of uncertainty, which may explain why the doctors delayed the decision. "I think candidly, because of my dad's position, they were reluctant to make the call until then," he says. "At the same time, they were concerned that the wall of the colon would perforate. It finally came to a point where they had no other choice. And in a way, I'm glad," Marvin adds. "Some people have an option, and consequently, don't pursue surgery because they're afraid. I didn't have a choice. It was either that or die."

Margaret still remembers the day the doctors told her they had scheduled emergency surgery for her husband. "It's the first and only time my knees gave way," she says. "I thought I was going to collapse. The whole thing was fast and furious. They didn't know what they'd find. They didn't know how bad the colitis was. It turned out to be much worse than they had predicted."

Mrs. Bush, who had only the day before left for Santa Fe, New Mexico, to help with a charity fundraiser, found herself urgently summoned back to Washington, having been told only that Marvin's vital signs were failing. "I tried to pretend that I wasn't afraid," she writes in her memoirs. "Nothing could happen to our precious boy. I was praying that he would be all right." Her biggest fear—that her husband would be at the steps of the plane when she arrived, which would indicate that Marvin didn't make it—went unrealized. Instead, she arrived at the hospital to find the Vice President "sitting at Marvin's bedside, with his hand on his arm." According to Margaret, it would not be the last time her father-in-law would be at Marvin's side in the ensuing weeks.

"I remember, after Marvin's surgery, his father would bring his briefcase and sit in the chair, in the corner with the light on, and spend hours there, quietly working," says George Bush's daughter-in-law. From the time she first met her future in-laws, she realized she was marrying into a warm, loving family who really cared for each other. "Of course, that was no small matter," she says. "It meant a plethora of Secret Service men and intense hospital security. It was a huge deal."

Marvin remembers little about those hours leading up to his surgery. He dimly recalls seeing "that famous white hair of my mother" and wondering what she was doing there. He has a vague recollection of the doctors pointing to his side and trying to explain what an ostomy was. Other than that, the memories of that time mingle together in an indistinct blur of days blending into weeks, weeks into months.

He did, however, sense that he was dying. Writes his

mother in her memoirs, "Marvin told me later that he thought he was dying when two things happened: His dad spent the day by his side, and his brother, Jeb, called just to pass the time of day. He ended his call with 'I love you, Marvin.' My boys don't say things like that to each other. They just know it and act it. That day, Jeb said it."

Marvin didn't die, but there were moments when he wished he had. He'd lost a significant amount of weight and was often in such terrible pain that he found himself begging for painkillers. All of this led to one nightmarish moment when an adverse reaction to morphine sent him into frenzied hallucinations. Horrified nurses found the newly sutured Marvin jumping out of bed, talking loudly, and yanking IV lines from his arm.

For Margaret, who had faced her own health challenges as a child, watching her husband go through the healing process brought back memories of when she was diagnosed with an extremely rare case of ovarian cancer at age five that left her unable to have children of her own. She came alongside her husband during those dark days, offering the kind of empathy only someone who's been through similar circumstances can offer. She also provided the strength he needed not only to endure the healing process, but to face the harsh reality of life with an ostomy, as well.

"We thought we were in the valley of the shadow of death," says Margaret. "None of us was sure he'd pull through."

Yet for every shadow, there are boundaries, and outside the boundaries, sunlight shining in all its dazzling brilliance. While Marvin was lying in a hospital in Washington that bleak and terrible month of May, unbeknownst to him, somewhere in the heart of Texas, on the outskirts of that shadow, a baby girl was being born.

An Important Phone Call

About a month after Marvin's surgery—weak, sore, and discouraged, but nevertheless needing to get back in circulation—Marvin sat in his office, trying to catch up with a backlog of work. It was June 1986—two days before Father's Day. His assistant walked in and said, "Marvin, you have a phone call. It's important. I think you should take it."

Marvin picked up the phone, and a woman's voice said, "Marvin, I want to wish you a happy Father's Day."

Marvin remembers thinking. *How cruel. Why would someone torment me like this?* But she said it again: "Happy Father's Day, Marvin."

It took a moment before he understood. He set the phone down and began to sob. It was the adoption agency, and they had a little girl that needed a home and a father and a mother.

The next day, he and Margaret stood in the waiting room of the Edna Gladney Home in Fort Worth, Texas. Cradled in his arms was his newborn daughter—four-week-old Marshall Lloyd Bush.

For Marvin, it was as if he had been nudged, at long last, out of the gloom and bleakness into the blinding brilliance of a new day and a new future—a future with hope and light that now included the little girl they were about to adopt.

The stepping stone before him was clear. He had work to do. Not what has been, but what will be—that's what mattered. Behind him lay the shadow; before him the sunshine and purpose, a reason for getting well. It was time to get strong again. Time to find the energy he would need—to be a dad.

Three years after they adopted Marshall, the Bushes adopted their second child, a little boy named Walker. On January 20, 1989, Marvin Bush stood with his wife on the steps of the White House and watched his father become the 41st President of the United States. Twelve years later, he would be there again, witnessing the inauguration of his older brother, George W. Bush.

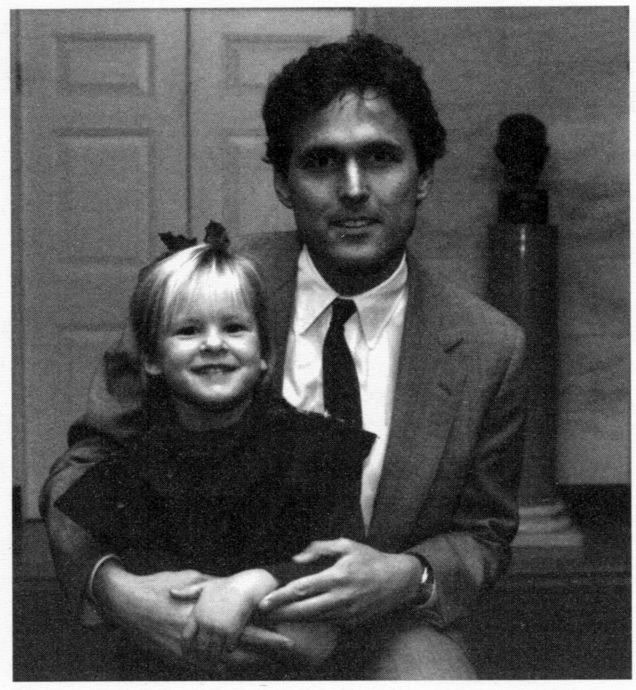

That's Marvin with his adopted daughter Marshall, who arrived just a few weeks after his surgery and helped turn a very dark time into one filled with hope and optimism. I have had the privilege of getting to know Marvin and his wife, Margaret, as well as former First Lady Barbara Bush.

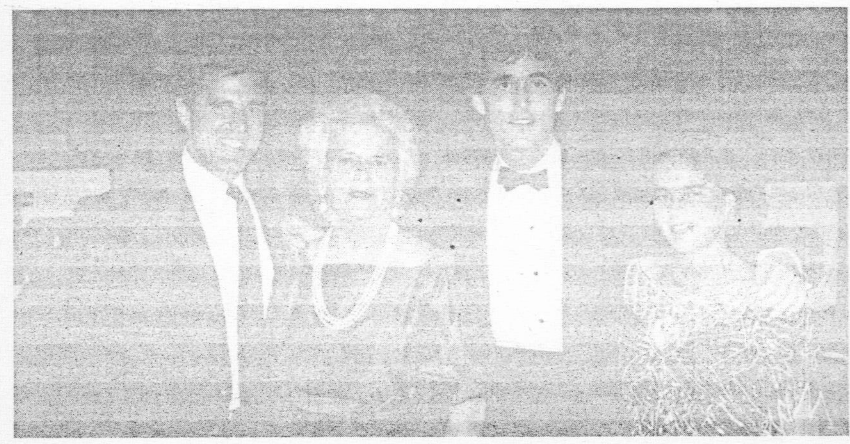

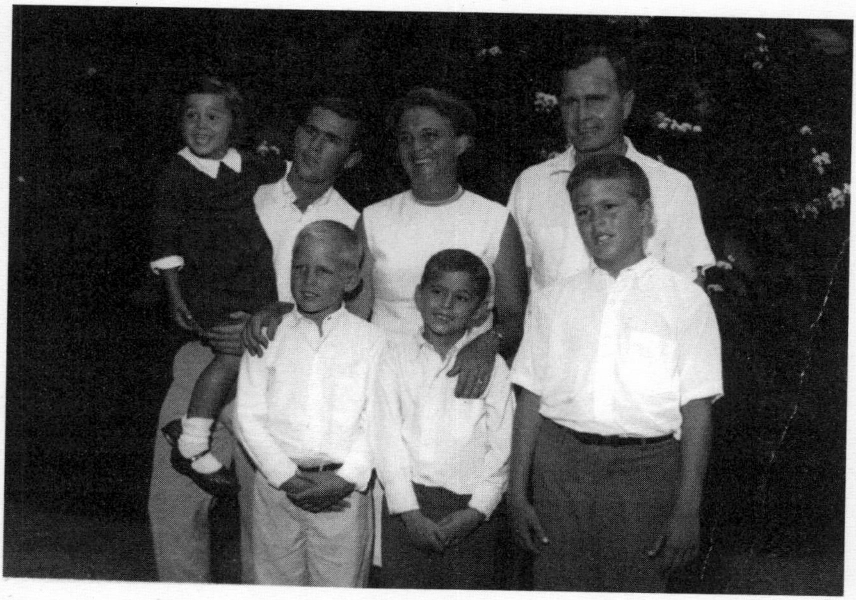

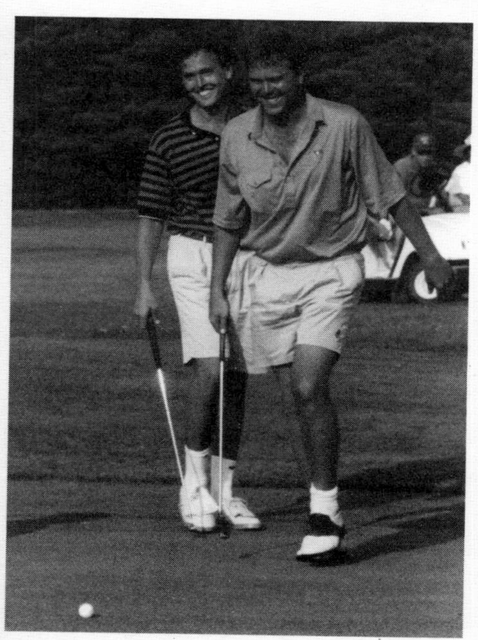

He's a President's son and a President's brother, but as Marvin Bush learned all too well, ulcerative colitis doesn't respect how famous your family is. Marvin is standing in the front center with his parents, George and Barbara, along with older brothers George W. and Jeb Bush.

In the midst of his father's political career, Marvin required ileostomy surgery at the age of twenty-nine, but he quickly resumed his athletic pursuits, including golfing with his brother, Jeb (left), and his first love, tennis.

When Life Deals You a Bad Hand

LUCY AMBROSI

AGE
34

HOMETOWN
Bethesda, Maryland

MEDICAL SITUATION
Symptomatic at the age of nine, diagnosed with IBD at thirteen, she endured twenty surgeries, culminating in a permanent ileostomy.

Right about the time most teenage girls are getting their drivers' permits and worrying about their first dates, Lucy Ambrosi had other things on her mind.

Like whether she would make it through fourth period without having to get up in the middle of American History and use the restroom for the third time that day.

Like whether one change of clothing in her backpack was enough, or if she would need two?

Like whether she should order cheese pizza like all her friends, or stick with something bland, like mashed potatoes.

Like whether she should eat anything at all, for that matter, since there was a basketball game that night.

Things like that.

More to the point, though, was the question of whether she would live to see another day. Especially that terrible night in 1983 when the fifteen-year-old woke up in such pain it was all she could do to bang on her bedroom wall and pray that someone would come and rescue her. Fortunately, her sister, Jorie, visiting for the weekend, was asleep in the room next door and woke up when she heard the racket.

Lucy's mother remembers that night as though it were yesterday. "It was her brother's birthday, and Lucy had been sitting across the table from me earlier in the evening," recalls Helen Koch, who at seventy-five has not relinquished her most cherished role in life as mom to her daughter. "She had on a pink angora sweater at the time, and I remember thinking how lovely she looked. But later on, in the middle of the night, we had to rush her to the hospital."

What happened, explains Lucy, is that her small intestine had perforated, allowing fecal matter to spill into the sterile sac surrounding her bowels. The resulting peritonitis would probably have killed her without radical medical intervention. After hastily consulting several surgeons, Lucy's parents signed the papers allowing doctors to perform a life-saving resection of Lucy's intestine.

Helen Koch says she and her husband were confident this nightmarish experience would put an end, once and for all, to the endless cycle of health problems their youngest daughter had experienced since she was a child.

Little did they know that Lucy's problems were only beginning.

An Insidious Disease

Lucy Ambrosi is the sixth and youngest child of George and Helen Koch (pronounced "Cook"). Though all the Koch children are bright and spirited, it was Lucy, the youngest, who emerged as the feistiest. From somewhere in her parents' gene pool, Lucy had inherited an indomitable will and a resolute invincibility. Unfortunately, Lucy also inherited something else—Crohn's disease, an "insidious disease that hops right along the digestive tract," as her mother puts it. Though Crohn's disease can sometimes be controlled with medication and at times even slip into remission (as it did for Lucy's uncle), Lucy's disease progressed into a severe case that refused to let up.

Lucy believes she began displaying symptoms of the disease as early as third grade, when bouts of diarrhea became more frequent. Determined to help, Lucy's parents began taking her from one doctor to the next, trying to get a fix on what was wrong. After being misdiagnosed with lactose intolerance by pediatric specialists, she learned from Dr. Gary Roggin, a gastroenterologist, that she probably had ulcerative colitis or Crohn's disease. For a few years, that's what Lucy's parents assumed was troubling their daughter. That was confirmed on that terrible night in the emergency room, when the doctors conclusively diagnosed her with Crohn's disease.

As a teenager, Lucy began to develop an analytical detachment from her body, intuitively sensing that if this was the hand she was dealt, she had better figure out how to play it. She learned the subtle nuances of her digestive system and became proficient at regulating her food intake. In order to live as "normal" a life as possible, she studied the best way to control her environment.

Loss of bowel control was a huge concern, especially during those crucial adolescent years when self-esteem and body image issues dictate almost every waking hour. Lucy discovered very early that in order to get through a day without humiliation, she would need to be prepared for an emergency. She began carrying an extra set of clothing to school every day. Her close circle of friends knew about Lucy's disease and did what they could to help her cope with it—from helping her get to a bathroom quickly to allowing her to drive on their outings as they got older. So supportive were Lucy's peers, in fact, that on the day of her high school graduation, when the class was posing for senior photos, Lucy suddenly had to dash to the bathroom. Her entire class sat down and refused to proceed without her.

Such was Lucy's existence, from early childhood to young adulthood: always searching for a bathroom. Usually making it, but sometimes missing. Changing from soiled clothes to clean. Becoming panicked on an airplane when a beverage cart was between her and the lavatory. "It became a way of life," says Lucy, who became so adept at managing her disease that she taught herself how to control her bowels simply by not eating. It was either that or become a recluse. "Whenever you eat, the process of peristalsis—where your intestines start to push your food along—begins immediately, so you learn to adapt. If I knew I was going somewhere where there would be no easy access to a toilet, I would skip a meal so I could make it through the evening."

That's not to say she didn't slip up now and again. "Being part Italian, it was so hard to pass up a good pizza," she acknowledges with a smile. "But when I ate pizza, I'd feel lousy afterward, but I would still go to school anyway."

When pressed, Lucy does admit that she felt lousy most of the time while growing up. According to her mother, however, she never complained. "It was always amazing to me," Helen says. "She was so sick for so many years. I used to wonder if deep down she ever questioned, 'Why me?' If she did, she never expressed it. She never let any of us feel sorry for her, and she certainly never let on that she felt sorry for herself. She'd just say, 'This is what life gave to me, and this is what I have to deal with.' "

Lucy counters by insisting she could never have gotten through her school years without the support of her parents. "My parents were my strongest advocates," says the energetic thirty-four-year-old nurse. "I was fortunate, not only to have a mother who was always around, but a dad who, in spite of his grueling work schedule, never missed a doctor's appointment and never once let me face a surgery alone—all twenty of them."

Chronic illness notwithstanding, Lucy managed to graduate from high school with good grades. And having attended a college-prep school where higher education is a given, the next logical step for the eighteen-year-old graduate was to do what every other kid does after graduation: move away from home and go to college. And that's exactly what Lucy decided to do.

The College Years

She was accepted at Denison University, a private college in Granville, Ohio, about forty-five miles outside of Columbus. The summer before her freshman year, Lucy and her entire extended family gathered at the Greenbrier Golf Resort in the Shenandoah Valley, where the Koch clan has vacationed every August since 1950. It was a huge gathering—Lucy's older siblings and their spouses and children, a few scattered relatives, and, of course, the grandparents. Lucy's parents had planned to drive to the university campus and get Lucy settled in her dorm after their vacation. No sooner had everyone settled in and unpacked for the two-week holiday, however, when the phone rang. It was Lucy's doctor. Lucy's red blood cell count was dangerously low. She was severely anemic and would need to return to Maryland as soon as possible for a blood transfusion.

Disappointed but not surprised—she'd come to accept detours as part of the package—she packed her things. To her dismay, however, so did everyone else. Her brother, Bobby, who shares the same blood type as Lucy, went along to do the transfusion. Her parents went because that's what her parents have done since Lucy was a girl. And everyone else? How could they stay? It just wouldn't be right. The vacation ended before it began. Lucy traveled to the hospital and received not only the transfusion, but an additional round of steroid treatments, as well.

The hospital diversion delayed her arrival at college, and Lucy sensed almost from the beginning that Denison wasn't the place for her. It was as though it wasn't meant to be. She had arrived at school three weeks late when the term was in full swing—relationships established, sororities rushing, and course work begun in earnest. Not only that, Lucy was so thin that the girls in the dorm room suspected she was anorexic. They began to whisper. If they only knew. When her weight dropped to eighty-five pounds, Lucy lost heart. She called her parents and said it was time to come home and get healthy again.

She then began to cycle through a spate of doctors, drugs, and therapy. She spent seven months eating no food and receiving high levels of essential nutrients—lipids, minerals, potassium, electrolytes—through a TPN (total parenteral nutrition) catheter inserted into to a large vein in her chest. Though she knew physically that her body was being nourished, the "fast" was difficult psychologically. "Eating is a big part of our life," explains Lucy. "I'd be hanging out with my family, and they'd be eating. It was hard not to eat when I saw how much they were enjoying the meal."

She tried to remain optimistic, and she certainly never complained. But gradually it dawned on her that this couldn't go on. Here she was, nearly twenty, and her life had degenerated to one of mere existence. She was literally shuffling through life from bathroom to bathroom. At some point during the seven-month "no eating" plan, a light bulb went on.

"It became clear to me that we were treating symptoms, not the disease," says Lucy, who by this time had taken an active role in her health, aggressively researching the disease and dialoguing with nurses and specialists. Knowing that she wanted to get married and have a family someday, she became terrified that she might be doing irreparable harm to her reproductive system, so she refused to take any more of the drugs the doctors were prescribing.

And so it came as no surprise to her parents when one afternoon Lucy stood in the kitchen of their house and said quietly, "I've decided. I want to have my colon out." Here's another moment seared forever in Helen's memory—as vivid today as it was that afternoon. "I can still remember where she was standing. I remember thinking, what a terribly courageous decision for a young person to make."

Once the decision was made, it was simply a matter of finding the right physician. With their shopping list of recommended surgeons in hand, the Kochs headed out the door, wisely allowing their strong-willed daughter to take the lead. Their search ended in the pristine office of Dr. Victor Fazio at the Cleveland Clinic. "I'd been to hundreds of doctor appointments to that point," Lucy explained, "so I had a pretty good idea of what I was looking for. Within ten minutes of meeting Dr. Fazio, I was ready to jump on the operating table. I had never been more ready to do anything."

She would gladly have undergone surgery that day, but Dr. Fazio recommended that she wait three months to give her body time to clear all the steroids from her system. Finally, in March 1988, Lucy Koch went under the surgeon's knife again—this time, voluntarily. Dr. Fazio removed her entire colon and rectum, as well as part of her small intestine, and created a permanent ileostomy.

When Lucy emerged from anesthesia, it was in the presence of her entire family—her parents and her sister and four brothers. "Waking up to all their faces is one of the most powerful and vivid memories of my lifetime," she says. "I don't think they realized how much they contributed to my strength each in a special way, whether it was humor, emotional support, protectiveness, or just a silent, yet safe presence. I knew I could get through anything with them there."

Her family had watched this beautiful and talented young woman endure the indignities and pain of a disease that is hard to talk about, let alone experience. They watched as she studied the swollen red stoma on her abdomen and the enormity of her decision swept over her in a mixture of both aversion and relief. Like the random flip of a card from a dealer's deck, they knew Lucy had been dealt a difficult hand. Nevertheless, they hoped this second surgery, as difficult and life-altering as it was, would put an end to the horrible experience that had made up most of Lucy's life.

Lay All the Cards on the Table

Several months after the surgery, Lucy was elated with the new lease on life she had received. Freed from the ball and chain of bathrooms and the unpredictability of her intestines, she felt good—and even went so far as to agree to a blind date with a handsome fellow her brother knew.

Lucy had made up her mind that whoever she dated, that person would have to accept her as she was—ostomy and all. Better to lay your cards on the table, she figured, than delay the inevitable. When she told her blind date about the pouch, to her surprise he was neither put off nor repulsed. If anything, he was curious.

"I knew a bit about her health problems and the ileostomy going into the relationship, but I didn't care," says Steve Ambrosi, who was working for Lucy's brother at the time. Immediately enamored by the vivacious, pretty, and eloquent woman sitting across the table from him, he plied her with questions, and she supplied the answers. "The ostomy didn't make a difference to me at all," he continues. "I wanted to know more about it so I could better understand what she was going through. She's a wealth of knowledge and was very clear in describing what was going on."

Steve and Lucy had been dating for only three months when Lucy was rushed back to the Cleveland Clinic, where she underwent her third major surgery, this time to repair a fistula next to her stoma. For many twenty-one-year-old men, this could have been a deal-breaker, but it wasn't. As she sensed when she met Steve, he showed nothing but care and compassion as he accompanied Lucy on the flight to Cleveland, and he was there at her side when she awoke from surgery.

Ask either of them if they think they've gotten a raw deal from life, and both Steve and Lucy seem almost baffled by the question. "This is just something we have to do," says the thirty-four-year-old regional director for Domino's Pizza. "When her disease flares up, we have to deal with it. That's part of our life. And who am I to complain? She's the one who has to suffer."

As for Lucy, she sees nothing but good in the "hand" she's been dealt. True, she struggled with infertility, the obvious consequence of a lifetime of powerful drugs, invasive surgeries, and the constant ravages of Crohn's disease. Both her first and second pregnancies were dangerously high risk, requiring a Terbutaline pump in her leg that administered a drug to keep her uterine contractions from becoming too frequent or too strong. She also had a Metaport surgically placed in her right atrium to infuse a high volume of fluid to maintain hydration, due to her short bowel syndrome.

Each pregnancy required Herculean efforts on her part since she was kept on bed rest at the Cleveland Clinic for four months each time, awaiting a C-section because she was told that there was no way she could have vaginal deliveries. "Under the close care of Dr.

Elliot Philipson at the Cleveland Clinic, we learned so much from the first pregnancy, and that really helped us manage the second pregnancy," says Lucy. "With my daughter Victoria, I was only able to make it to thirty-four weeks, but with my second pregnancy, my son, Stephen, was born at thirty-seven weeks. We are so fortunate today to be blessed with two healthy and happy children."

No Big Deal

Although Lucy has been sidetracked a dozen times and been denied what most would consider a "normal" childhood and adolescence, she doesn't think that life has given her a raw deal. She has lived with pain so long now she hardly gives it a second thought.

Tucked somewhere in that bad hand she was dealt long ago is an ace of spades. It was sometime in the fall of 1990 that Lucy decided to go into nursing. She graduated from the Georgetown University Nursing School and went on to train as an Enterostomal Therapy nurse at the Cleveland Clinic under the supervision of the very nurses who tended to her during twenty surgeries. Caring for patients who have endured chronic illness, pain, and ostomy surgery has become a passion in her life, but the love of her life is caring for two miracle children. Her three-year-old daughter, Victoria, is named for Lucy's incredible surgeon, Dr. Victor Fazio, and her infant son is named for his proud Daddy.

The way Lucy sees it, she's just getting started. Some day, she would like six children, just like her parents. That is, if her doctors will let her.

Knowing Lucy, they will.

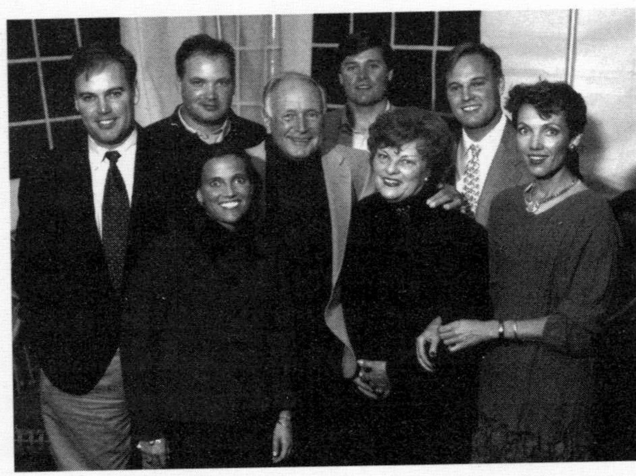

You won't find too many people with more spunk and determination than Lucy Ambrosi, who battled through a long and difficult battle with Crohn's disease in her teen years before her small intestine perforated and she required ileostomy surgery. She says it was her family that was always there before and after surgery that provided the support and encouragement she needed during those dark years.

Her husband, Steve, pictured here on their wedding day, stood by Lucy during all of her surgeries.

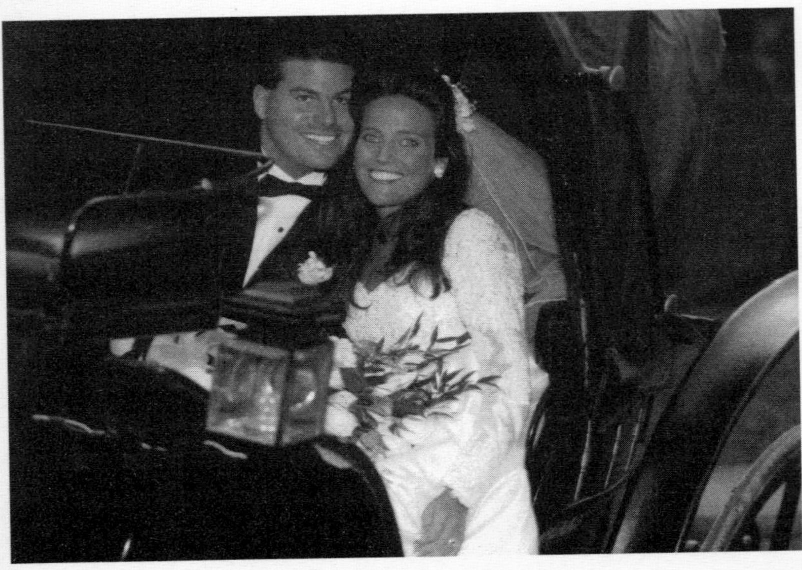

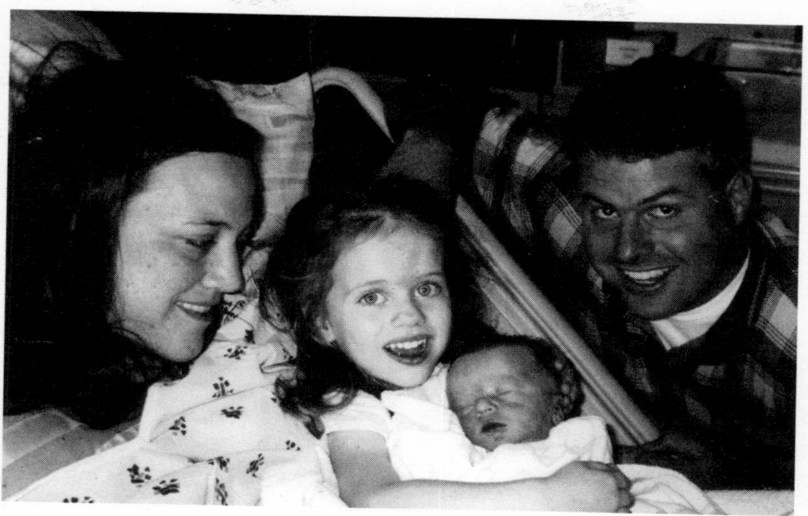

Today, Lucy is the proud mother of two children, Victoria and Stephen, both born after her ileostomy surgery and at the Cleveland Clinic, the same hospital where Dr. Vic Fazio performed her operation.

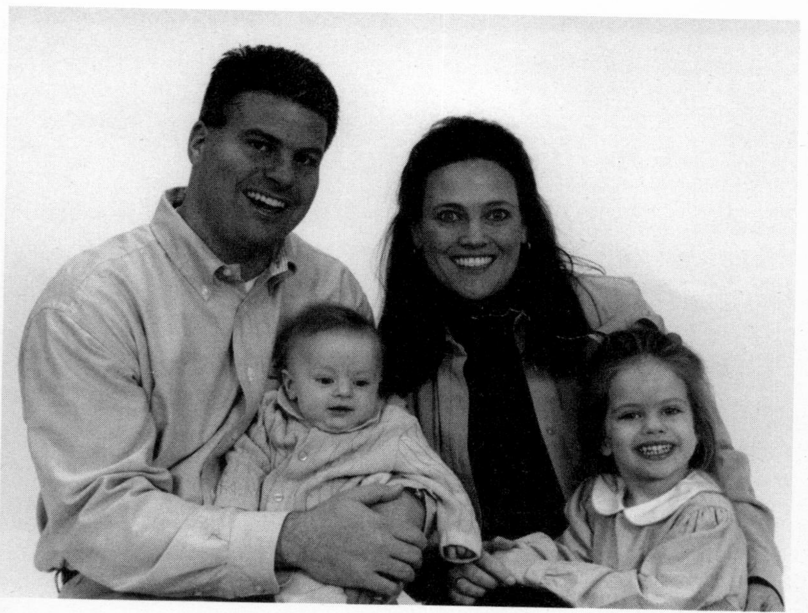

This Evil Thing

DAVE ALBERGA

AGE
39

HOMETOWN
La Jolla, California

MEDICAL SITUATION
Diagnosed with ulcerative colitis while attending West Point, he fought the disease for twenty years before needing an ileostomy that he eventually converted to a J-pouch.

Ask Dave Alberga what "normal" means, and he'll tell you that it's a cross between sailing, diving, and competing in triathlons. Here's someone who prefers climbing a lofty mountain summit to sitting in a comfortable armchair by a fire. Not your ordinary guy.

Which is why, when well-meaning doctors tried to assure Dave that he would be able to resume a "normal" life after colostomy surgery, it was about the worst thing they could tell him. "Their assessment of normal and my assessment of normal were two different things," says Dave, who is president and CEO of The Active Network, one of the leading providers of online registration and data management services for individual and participatory sports in the world. "I didn't want to live a 'normal' life. The idea terrified me." Unfortunately for Dave, his options were running out. The only reason surgery was being mentioned was because all other methods of dealing with his disease were no longer working.

Dave Alberga had lived nearly twenty years with ulcerative colitis. Twenty years spent always knowing where the nearest toilet was or carrying around an extra pair of under shorts, just in case. "I'd walk to work, soil my pants, walk home, change, walk back," he says, marveling in retrospect how it was he came to accept the gradual deterioration of his health with such equanimity. "It's like the proverbial frog in a pot of water that's slowly beginning to boil," he explains. "Over the course of years you grow so accustomed to the disease, you gradually adapt to it. You aren't even aware of how compromised your life has become."

Even Dave's wife, Christine, was baffled by Dave's tolerance of the disease when she and Dave first started dating. "I couldn't believe how much he put up with," says Christine, who met Dave in 1987 when the two of them worked for Procter & Gamble. "He didn't even make an effort to see a doctor. I couldn't understand that. In my way of thinking, when you're sick, you go to the doctor. Dave didn't think that way."

What Chris didn't know at the time was that Dave had seen doctors for his colitis, but the experience had rendered him skeptical of the process. Before he worked for Procter & Gamble, Dave had been an infantry officer in the U.S. Army. "I graduated from West Point Military Academy in 1984," he says, "and I went straight into the army, colitis and all. I graduated, got my degree, and then, because I was in such good physical shape, I managed to get a medical waiver in order to enter the infantry."

In spite of the waiver, it soon became obvious that Dave's illness would eventually thwart his military ambitions. Within a year after leaving West Point, he realized he couldn't handle the physically demanding lifestyle of an infantry officer with the disease. "I was losing a lot of blood," he says. "I was anemic, fatigued, losing weight. The disease had obviously compromised me."

After one particularly difficult flare-up, Dave admitted himself into an army hospital and learned first-hand the difference between military and civilian medicine: he underwent a full colonoscopy with no sedation. It was, to put it mildly, "pretty rough." After fewer than two years in the military, Dave received a medical discharge. Ulcerative colitis had dealt its first blow, and Dave was devastated.

"For the first time, I felt like I couldn't fight this thing any more," he recalls. "Until then, the disease had never prevented me from doing whatever I wanted to do. Yet here I was, sitting in the officers' quarters, waiting to be discharged, and wondering what I was going to do next. I hadn't thought about a civilian life. I felt like I'd failed."

Lots of Work and Play

Failure isn't a word that comes easily to Dave Alberga. Born in Putnam Valley, New York, Dave grew up in a household where children were expected to excel, no questions asked. The younger of two children, Dave did exactly that. In high school, he competed in sports—lacrosse, soccer, and track—and eventually graduated in the top of his class. "There was this expectation," he says. "It didn't matter what else I did: homework had to get done, and there had to be good report cards."

That's not to say Dave's childhood was all work and no play. On the contrary, the Albergas seemed to take play as seriously as they did work. "What was unusual about my family," Dave says, "is that every summer we'd travel. I'm not talking about going to Disneyland or Niagara Falls. I'm talking about extraordinary travel. I've been to about fifty countries in my life. One summer we spent nine weeks in the African bush. Another time we went to Europe where we bought a car and traveled the continent. One year we pitched a tent in the Adirondacks, and another we traveled 10,000 miles throughout the U.S. and Canada. I'd been to Iran, India, Turkey, Poland, Czechoslovakia—you name it—by the time I graduated from high school."

Growing up in such a well-traveled family, Dave entered adulthood with the mindset that nothing was insurmountable. To him, obstacles merely represented challenges to overcome. Indeed, Dave seemed to welcome challenges, which no doubt accounts for why he opted for the West Point Military Academy over the objections of his parents. "Part of my going to the Academy was youthful rebellion," Dave admits. "My parents probably would have preferred something less rigid and oppressive for their son."

It was during Dave's junior year at West Point that his colitis was first diagnosed. "My first symptoms were diarrhea, blood, some mucous," he says. "Nothing I couldn't handle. I did lose a lot of weight that third year, but I was able to push through. In fact, I was able to convince the U.S. Army that I was well enough for them to issue me a medical waiver."

As it turned out, well enough was not good enough. So it was, two years later, Dave found himself dressed in civilian clothes, living back home with his parents in New York, biding his time substitute teaching calculus and math at the high school where his mother taught. He did this for eight months until, in a combination of good luck and good timing, he landed a low-level job with Procter & Gamble in brand management, working on Maxi Pads and facial tissue business. He moved to the company headquarters in Cincinnati in 1987 and spent three years working for P&G, but he was sick and struggling the entire time.

Right about then, Christine Cernosia had just finished her undergraduate work at Colgate University. She was ready to celebrate. “My sister and I decided to throw a dinner party,” says Christine, who was working in the Systems Applications department at Procter & Gamble at the time. “We invited a few friends we both knew, but we needed one more person. I remembered this guy I’d just met in the office. He was cute, funny, and very smart. Interestingly, my sister had just met him that same day as well. We decided to give him a call.”

Meanwhile, unbeknownst to Chris, Dave was talking to people at work about “the greatest woman” he’d just met and was wondering how to snag a date with her. In the middle of his conversation, the phone rang. It was Christine. When he was finished talking with her, he hung up the phone and grinned proudly at his colleagues. “That was Christine, and she just asked me out to a dinner party.”

Christine laughs when she hears the story. “It was as if he thought he’d already done his magic on this young girl,” she says. They became friends quickly though, and after four months they began dating seriously. “We tried to take things slowly, since we were both coming out of other relationships,” Christine remembers, “but we had so much fun together that we decided to just go with it and see what happened."

Dave's colitis was no secret, and it was Christine who finally convinced him to see a doctor. "Dave's the kind of guy who has a hard time admitting that he needs help. For him, there's a feeling that you should be able to handle things on your own. For a long time, Dave had coped with the symptoms and the discomfort of his disease by self-medicating and by sheer determination. What he didn't recognize, though, was how much he was changing his life for the colitis. Even though he wasn't debilitated, he was making too many concessions to the disease." Once Dave agreed to see a doctor, however, a huge hurdle was cleared.

It wasn't long before Cincinnati began to feel too small for Dave and Christine. Ready to further their education but not ready to be apart, they applied to and were both accepted to graduate school at Stanford University. They recall their Stanford years in Palo Alto as among their best. Dave's disease seemed to stabilize, and he was among like-minded peers. In the best physical shape since he'd been in the military, he and Chris began doing high-altitude mountaineering and mountain biking. He felt like he was back, doing the things he loved, and no longer compromised by the disease.

The hallmark of these years for Dave was climbing the 14,496-foot tall Mt. Whitney, the Central California peak that is the tallest mountain in the contiguous United States. "The Whitney climb was a benchmark for me," he says. "We chose a reasonably difficult route, a three-day climb, with steep rock and ice. There were six of us, but only Christine and I and one other person reached the summit. It was a fantastic climb, and it galvanized me. From that point forward, we did a couple of climbs a year." For Dave, his battle with colitis seemed like a thing of the past.

A Chance to Go Down Under

Shortly before they married in 1991, however, the disease dealt its second major blow. Fresh out of graduate school and armed with two Masters degrees, Dave was offered a job in Sydney, Australia, with the Boston Consulting Group, an international strategy and management consulting firm. "The job matched my qualifications perfectly," says Dave. Optimistic, Dave and Chris packed their apartment and hammered out their future plans.

Then came the blow. Concerned that Dave might become a medical liability on their socialized medicine plan, the Australian government turned down his application for a work visa. For a second time, the disease had thwarted his ambitions, and for a second time, Dave was devastated. They appealed to the Australian government while spending their honeymoon at Chris's parents' house in Detroit. When Australia failed to reverse its decision, Dave went to work for the Boston Consulting Group in Chicago. After eighteen months and two bitter Midwest winters, they decided to return to the West Coast, where Dave's entrepreneurial career began to take off.

At Christine's urging, Dave started training for triathlons, a grueling, three-event race that typically involves a one-mile swim, a twenty-five-mile bike ride, and a six- to twelve-mile run. Dave never considered himself to be a great endurance athlete, and he certainly never favored running. Not one to spurn a challenge, however, he trained aggressively, and in August 1999, he and Christine participated in the Hood to Coast two-hundred and five-mile-mile relay race that began in Portland, Oregon. According to Christine, Dave's best leg of the relay was running seven miles at 2:00 a.m. in pitch dark. Dave was hooked.

But his colitis wouldn't go away, and the disease struck its third and final blow in September 2000, when Dave was thirty-eight. Until then, the symptoms had been relatively minor and sporadic. Dave would treat them for a few months, wean himself of whatever medication he was taking, and then forge ahead. In September, however, he came down with the stomach flu. He assumed he'd be down for a day or so and then get back on his feet. After a few days, though, the colitis broadsided him. He began hemorrhaging, losing "a shocking amount of blood" every time he used the toilet. He was admitted to the hospital, where the doctors recommended high doses of steroids to calm the inflammation.

Dave's first hospital stay lasted four days. Seemingly better, he went home, hoping to ride it out. Within days, however, he was back. As Chris tells it, Dave was filling the toilet with blood and almost passing out in the bathroom. Until then, surgery had never been discussed. It was apparent to Chris, however, that the disease had spiraled out of control and other options had to be considered. She began to take charge.

"Dave was always the rock in our relationship," says Chris. "I'm more emotional. But when Dave got sick in September, I became the rock. I began researching every doctor and every treatment. I called perfect strangers in the middle of the night asking for advice and learning as much as I could. During the day I'd stay on top of the nurses, demand medications, and learn the benefits and side effects of the long list of medications. Every patient needs a strong advocate. I don't know how people go through this without someone at their side but they do. People kept asking me how I could do everything while keeping myself together, but there was no choice. This was my job. All that mattered was getting Dave better."

One thing that puzzled Dave and Chris was "Why now? Why was the disease so out of control after twenty years? Dave was only thirty-eight years old, too young for such a surgery." After talking to several doctors and patients, Dave and Chris learned that the average age for someone facing surgery for colitis is somewhere between the ages of twenty-two and forty.

When the subject of surgery came up, Dave refused to listen. "Everyone kept telling him that he'd feel better after the surgery," Chris recalls. "But how can you tell someone to submit to this kind of an operation? I've had major knee surgery before, but knee surgery is not the same as having a major organ removed."

Dave admits that things had to get pretty bad before he would finally consider the possibility of surgery. "I tried to hang on for as long as I could because I had so much fear," he explains. "I don't consider my activity level to be normal, and I felt like life wouldn't be worth living if I had to reduce it. So far, I hadn't met anyone who could say, 'I've lived a pretty extraordinary life, in spite of the surgery.' I needed to talk with people like me."

"Dave kept saying no one understood what he was going through," Chris recalls.

So, out of desperation, Chris began searching out people who had been through this kind of surgery and gone on to live extraordinary lives.

"I had a hard time giving him any perspective since I wasn't the one who was facing surgery. But when he was finally able to read about and speak with other people who were like him, Dave agreed to go ahead with the surgery. When he did, it was like a gigantic weight was lifted from his shoulders."

A Horrifying Condition

The decision came none too soon. After several transfusions and a roller coaster of results from mega dosages of steroids, Dave went into surgery in November 2000 weighing one hundred and thirty-seven pounds with a hematocrit level of twenty-four, nearly half the normal level. The doctor who operated on him was horrified by his condition. " I thought I'd seen it all, but Dave had the worse colon I've ever seen," said the doctor.

Because he had waited so long, recovery was complicated and potentially life-threatening. His heart rate skyrocketed; his hemoglobin levels dropped; and he continued to require several blood transfusions. Though Chris never thought she would lose him—"he's a real fighter"—the doctors were concerned. In retrospect, seeing how difficult his recovery was, both Chris and Dave realize now how unwise it had been to wait so long for surgery. "It's a huge, life-changing decision," Chris says, "but seeing all that Dave went through, I would recommend that people not wait. Complications can arise, and the recovery process can be much more difficult."

For Dave, surgery was more than a medical decision. It represented conquest of an insidious foe that had knocked him down one time too many. When his colon came out, it was as if he had purged himself of "this evil thing."

That's not to say he relished the idea of life with an ostomy. Filled at first with self-pity and revulsion, he felt "inhuman—like an animal." Nevertheless, he approached his recovery much the same as he approaches anything in life: a challenge. He learned that there was a triathlon scheduled in May 2001, and he set his sights on that. "It was training with a twist," he jokes. "I couldn't climb the stairs, let alone go out for a run. Yet here I was, signing on for a triathlon."

With the help of good friends and family and a never-say-die mindset that had served him well, six months after undergoing major abdominal surgery and wearing an ileostomy appliance, Dave Alberga finished the Mission Bay Spring Sprint. "We weren't fast," he says with a grin, "but we weren't last, either." Even friend and fellow triathlete Jon Belmonte marvels at Dave's accomplishment. "I can't believe he ran this thing with the equivalent of a gunshot wound in his side," he said after the race. "It was remarkable to see."

Why did he do it? Dave shrugs. "It was personally satisfying, knowing I could overcome what seemed like insurmountable odds." He pauses, then adds, "That's not completely true. I also wanted to show people that ostomy surgery doesn't have to slow you down. It doesn't have to be a life-ending thing. That's why I race."

Dave returned to the hospital at the end of May for follow-up surgery, this time to reverse the ileostomy and receive what Chris and Dave jokingly refer to as "modified plumbing"—a J-pouch. Two months later, Dave was back on his bike, swimming laps, and going on hour-long runs, training for the next triathlon.

In other words, everything was back to normal.

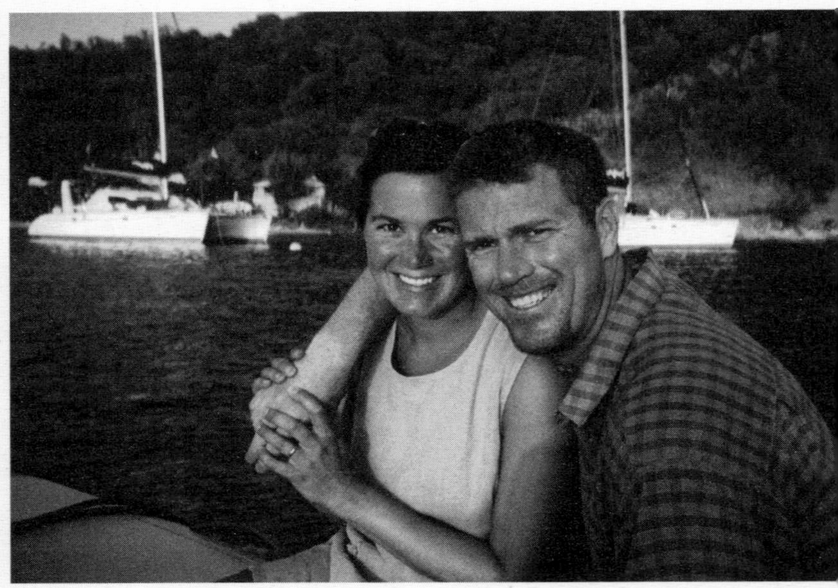

Dave Alberga has always seen the glass as half full, even though he lived for nearly twenty years with his illness before needing an ileostomy.

His wife, Christine, who married Dave in the middle of his battle with ulcerative colitis, was amazed at how much he endured before finally submitting to surgery.

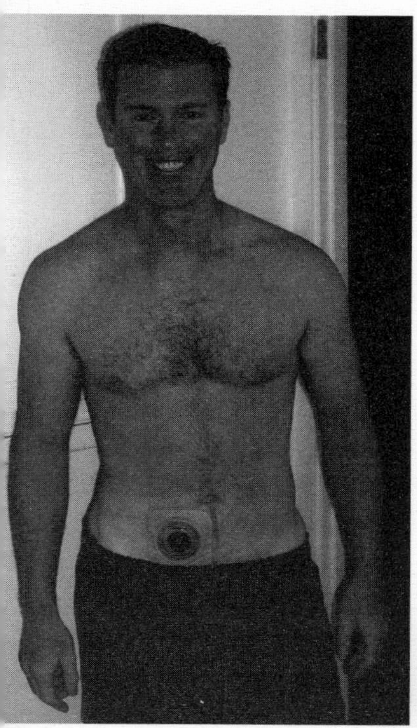

Dave proudly displays his stoma shortly before competing in—and completing—a mini-triathlon only six months after his surgery.

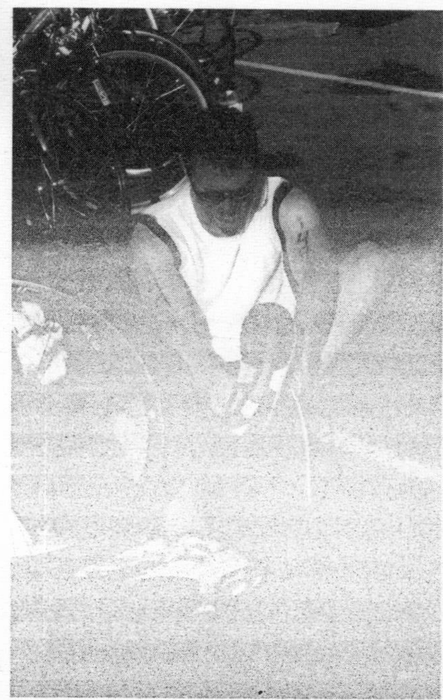

Faith Over Fear

LIZA FRAMPTON

AGE

43

HOMETOWN

Encinitas, California

MEDICAL SITUATION

At the age of forty, Liza began experiencing unexplained anemia, which led to the discovery of cancer and the need for subsequent ileostomy surgery.

The water flowing into the Pacific Ocean from Batiquitos Lagoon is calm on this May afternoon, and the skies are unseasonably overcast. Sea gulls and pelicans dive for meals, and an alert observer might glimpse a fish breaking the surface of the Carlsbad lagoon—a leap, a splash, and a ripple. To the west, a small mountain stands sentinel, its summit just visible through the clouds.

Liza Frampton has hiked the trails surrounding this lagoon many times. Today, her six-year-old daughter, Kate, rides piggyback, skinny legs wrapped around her mother's waist, arms clinging to her neck, an impish grin on her face. After a few paces, she slides to the ground and scampers up a hill. Liza laughs and follows, then stops to point to the peak.

"That's the mountain I had in my mind," she explains, pausing to catch her breath. "It reminded me of heaven. Always there, never changing. I kept my eyes on it while all these bad things kept happening to me."

From the top of a hill, Kate shouts and Liza resumes her climb. This forty-three-year-old mother of two daughters looks strong—happy and content. She greets fellow hikers with a wave, her stride long, her steps sure, and her arms swinging rhythmically. Auburn hair, wavy and cut short, frames an attractive face, highlighted by hazel eyes, a heart-shaped mouth quick to smile, and glossy white teeth that would make any dentist proud. Liza smiles a lot, as though life is the most delightful thing. Nothing—not a cloud nor a sigh—has ever dampened her cheerful spirit.

Life may be the most delightful thing to Liza, but her life has been anything but sunny. In fact, those who know her say she really shouldn't even be here today. Says one friend, "If you saw what I saw in that hospital, you'd agree. Liza's a living miracle."

A self-described "go-getter," Liza Frampton was born and raised in Honolulu, Hawaii, and lived there through most of her early teen years before moving back to the Mainland in the early '70s. Both of Liza's parents were very successful—her father was an attorney and her mother was a high-profile fashion model who graced the pages of *Vogue* and *Ladies Home Journal* and flaunted the designs of Yves St. Laurent and Pierre Cardin. It was her mother who instilled in Liza an appreciation for appearances. "She was trim and beautiful, and I wanted to be like her," Liza muses. "So I exercised a lot and wore stylish clothes. Clothes were a huge part of my life."

Liza's childhood years in Hawaii were happy and idyllic—"We went to school barefoot!" she says—but even paradise has its dirty laundry, and Liza's family was no exception. At fifteen, Liza's parents divorced. A year later, her mother remarried a college sweetheart and life would never be the same.

"I remember coming home from school one day," Liza recalls, "and being told to pack for a special, surprise two-week vacation. My younger brothers and sister and I packed some things, and in the middle of the night we went to the airport and caught a plane. We were airborne when my mother dropped the bombshell. It wasn't a vacation at all. We were moving to Oklahoma City. I can still hear my ten-year-old sister screaming, crying for her daddy."

The eldest of four, Liza dealt with the divorce and the move differently. "Basically, I stuffed it," she says. "I put on a happy face and thought, *We can let this be an adventure*. I handled it, but I didn't really deal with my feelings."

By the time Liza entered college, she had targeted broadcast journalism as a career choice, first studying at Stephens College in Missouri, then transferring to Southern Methodist University in Dallas, Texas, where her budding broadcast career took off. She worked at several TV and radio stations, writing news stories, lugging cameras around, and learning all aspects of television news. She also did traffic reports while still in college, flying over Dallas in a single-engine plane and occasionally swooping down near the fraternity houses to drop donuts on the guys below.

When Liza's mother developed breast cancer during this time, true to form, Liza took charge. "I did everything I could to help my mom beat this thing," she says. "I tried to get her to change her diet. I bought her self-help tapes. I believed I could help make everything okay." Liza and her younger sister became their mother's primary caregivers, and it was during this seven-year period leading up to her mother's death that Liza got the sense she wasn't in charge. "I really thought I could cure her," she says. "When Mom died on my twenty-eighth birthday, it was as though God called me on the phone and said, 'Liza, you're not the one in control.' "

It took one more "phone call" before Liza finally got the message. As an up-and-coming television journalist doing investigative health and consumer reporting, anchoring the evening news, and hosting a live radio call-in show, Liza epitomized the enviable, have-it-all modern woman of the '90s. Now married to Jack Frampton, a commercial real estate broker in Dallas, and the mother of a newborn girl, Liza was hitting her stride in the world of broadcasting. Her next stop, she felt, was doing network news in New York.

Then the baby got sick. Six weeks after Kalli was born, with Jack away on business, Liza found herself maintaining bedside vigils at the hospital, desperately trying to will this tiny infant well. With each blood test and every shriek and wail, Liza agonized—wishing, wanting, and praying that she could take her baby's pain upon herself. On the fourth night, her mother-in-law took over the vigil to give her some rest. Liza went home and fell to her knees. Acutely aware that she was not at the helm, she surrendered herself to God. That night, as Liza relinquished control of her life, she had a profound sense that all would be well, even if the baby died.

Kalli didn't die. But now, God finally had Liza's attention.

It was during this time, while researching a story for her TV station, that Liza was exposed for the first time to a health condition that she had been unaware of. "I met a man who was in the business of marketing medical appliances for people who had had ostomy surgeries," she says. "I knew next to nothing about ostomies and didn't really want to learn about them, even from a professional standpoint. My gut reaction was, 'No thanks—let's not go there.' "

Not long after this seemingly irrelevant incident, a tantalizing job offer from a Los Angeles TV station lured the Framptons to Southern California. Liza's stint at the L.A. station lasted only a year. While it might be tempting to blame the producer, politics, or even personalities for her departure, Liza sees what happened next in her life from the perspective of faith. "God had given me a wake-up call when my mom died," she says. "Maybe I heard, but I didn't listen. When Kalli nearly died, I got another wake-up call. That time, I was listening. And so, when everything fell apart at KCAL TV, I knew it was God, trying to get my attention again."

Liza sensed the time had come to stop working. "Liza, go home," is how she puts it. The decision wasn't easy, for several reasons. This eldest daughter of two highly successful parents had inherited the same internal drive to excel. Exiting a fast-lane profession went against all her natural instincts. Then there were the finances to consider. Liza's career brought in a hefty paycheck, and losing it meant that the financial burden fell on Jack's shoulders. After lots of prayer and discussion, both agreed that it was best for Liza to leave her broadcasting job and for the young family to relocate to San Diego.

Little did they know God was not through "calling." During the summer of 1998 at the age of forty, Liza became sick, developing severe anemia and struggling with bowel and stool problems. She spent the summer visiting one doctor after another, submitting to invasive biopsies, rectal exams, colonoscopies, and blood tests, trying to discover what was going on. In August, she received her answer. An orange-sized tumor, located in Liza's rectal area and attached to her lower backbone, was almost completely blocking her rectum. The diagnosis: squamous cell carcinoma, a cancer often found in the anus area.

How close Liza came to dying isn't clear, but the doctors immediately recommended aggressive radiation and chemotherapy. The tumor responded well to the treatment, but in order to ensure complete removal, Liza found herself back in the hospital four months later. She would undergo complicated surgery that involved the complete resection of her rectum as well as the partial removal of her tailbone where the tumor had attached. It was a painful ordeal, but just the beginning.

Five years after competing with the best of the best in the limelight of television news reporting, Liza now lay in agony on a hospital bed, barely able to walk, her insides truncated, her intestines lacerated, and her internal tissues horribly radiated. But there was more to come. With the surgery came abscesses, infection, drainage catheters—and more surgery. This time, a diverting ileostomy was performed. Even with her faith intact, this final humiliation seemed more than she could bear.

"The first thing I remember," she recalls, "is being in the hospital bed, lying down, propped up, and this nurse fiddling with something on my abdomen. She was chatting and laughing and I remember thinking, *What are you so darned happy about?* Then I looked down at my stomach and I saw the stoma, and a wave of nausea passed over me. I gagged, literally, which is surprising, since as a health reporter I've pretty much seen it all. But somehow, this was different. It was me."

What Liza remembers most is the rage. All her life, beauty, clothing and appearance had been an integral part of both her personal and professional identity. Now, as she looked at herself with her small intestine protruding from her abdomen and an unsightly bag collecting her waste, she felt dirty and disgusted. "I was so ashamed," she says. "Almost like I had been sexually violated."

The nurses in the hospital taught her the mechanics of changing her ostomy appliance, but Liza wasn't ready. "I was in so much pain from cancer complications," she remembers. "I physically and emotionally just couldn't deal with it all."

That's when Jack stepped in. Undaunted by the magnitude of the situation and the weight of responsibility he now felt for Liza and the family—and buoyed by a renewed faith of his own—Jack rose to the occasion. He administered to Liza's bandages, flushed her drainage tubes, and changed her ileostomy appliances weekly. He fed the kids, did their schoolwork with them, and tended to many of the other issues related to a house with a seriously ill mom.

Although it took about a year, Liza now has the hang of her ileostomy. She empties her pouch many times during the day, sometimes irritated by the inconvenience of having to "go" so often, but she is thankful to be alive again and be an active mom in her daughters' lives.

Kalli, a bright and talented third-grader, struggles with health problems of her own and has had to endure insensitive comments from playmates who casually wonder when her mom's going to die. Her sister, six-year old Kate, copes better now, but for a long time she was afraid—and angry. "There was a time when she'd play with her dolls or her Beanie Babies, but they never had mommies," Liza recalls sadly. "I felt so responsible, especially because I could remember so vividly watching my own mother die. The hardest part of all this was letting go and trusting God with my children. There were times I was almost paralyzed with fear and sadness for them, and yet, in so many ways, it was my children who kept me going."

And that mountain. During the darkest times, after she first learned of her cancer and began enduring radiation treatments. When her hair fell out in clumps and she stopped menstruating, causing Liza to lose all hope of having any more children. When the pain in her back was like knives stabbing from the inside out; and lying still for a CAT scan was almost impossible because of the excruciating pain. When fistulas began to fester and ooze and her own waste seeped into her body, poisoning her system, and the only way she could endure another agonizing steroid injection was by gripping a friend's hands and focusing intently on her eyes. When her daughter drew a picture of a little girl with huge tears rolling down her face and a lightning bolt piercing her stomach. When she felt she was drowning, tumbling, perishing, out of control in raging, icy rapids—that's when she saw the mountain, reminding her of God, standing immovable, unchanging, fixed. That's what got her through.

At times, she admits, she still grows discouraged.

"There's a lot going on in my life I don't like," she says. "Right now, my husband is out of a job. We're moving into our seventh little rental house in ten years. I have a lot of down times. But when I cry out to God, I'm always comforted. Even as my battle continues, I believe God's promises. And sometimes, when I'm all alone, and needing to feel close to God, I turn on my favorite music, and I dance with Him. I can feel His heartbeat. I can feel mine. They're in sync. That's all I want—a heart that beats to the same rhythm as my Father in heaven."

Holding out her arms in a graceful curtsy to demonstrate, she lifts her face upward and smiles with sheer rapture. Then she steps forward—lithe, agile, and elegant. And she dances having now overcome her fears.

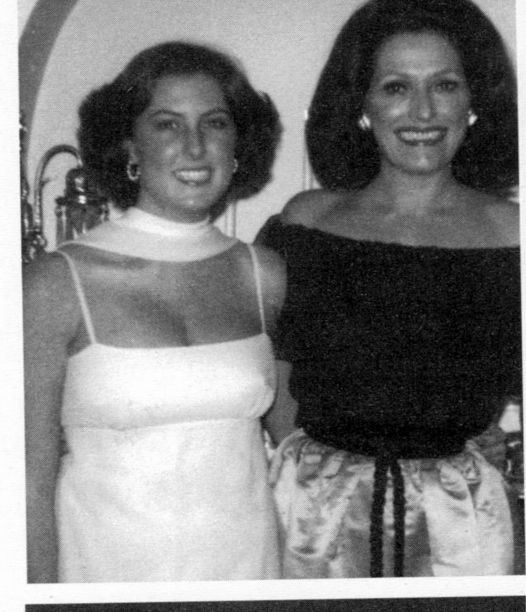

As a young woman, Liza Frampton learned style and grace from her mother.

After graduating from college, she became a news anchor in Dallas (that's her publicity photo) and an investigative television journalist specializing in health and consumer reporting.

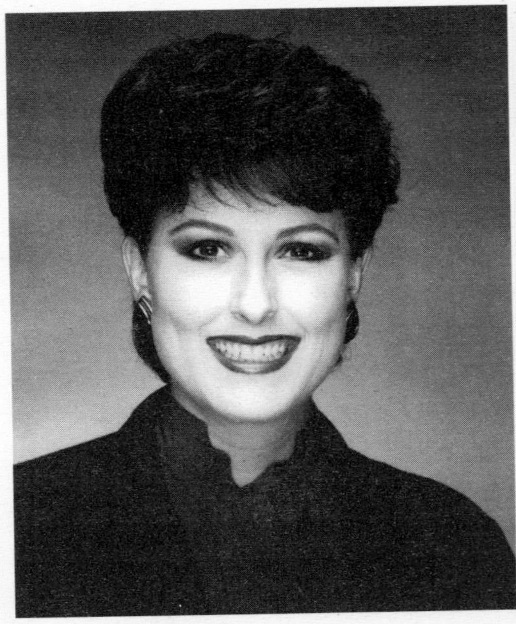

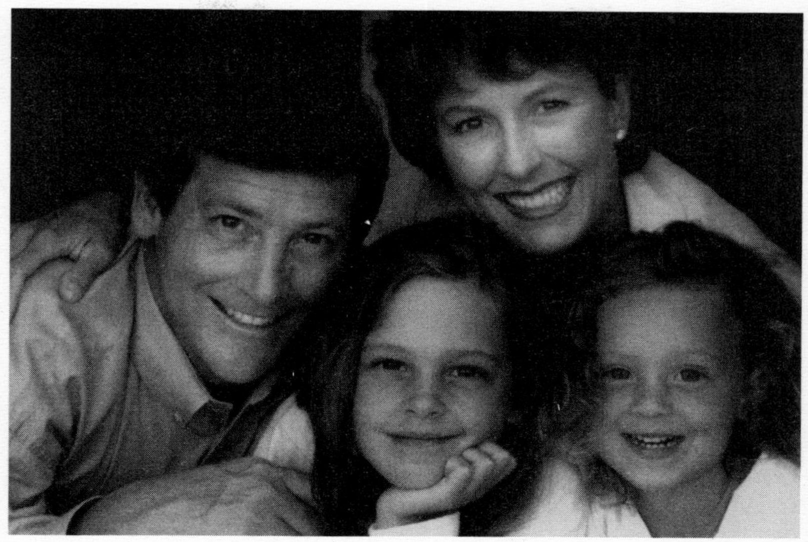

Liza decided to step away from the long hours of the television business to raise her two daughters, Kalli and Kate, and be home for her husband, Jack.

Unfortunately, her life was turned upside down when she was diagnosed with a cancerous tumor in her rectum that required radiation and chemotherapy. The difficult treatment caused her to lose her hair and almost her life, and in the end, left her with an ileostomy.

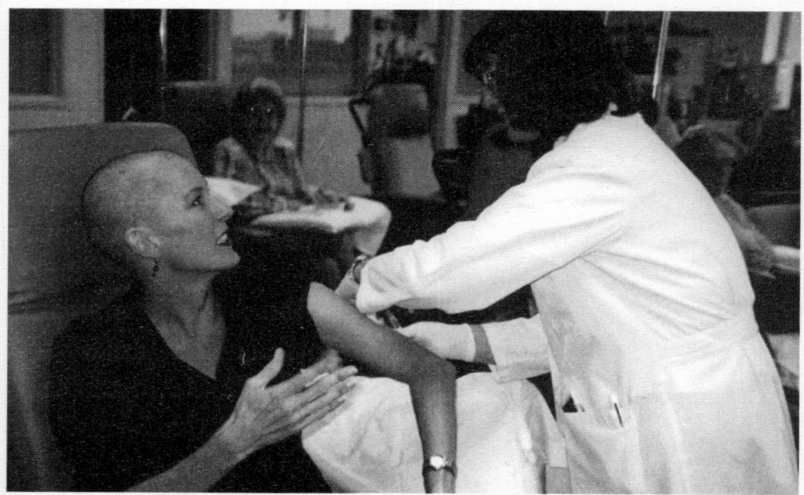

The Other Side of the Lens

BRIAN SISSELMAN

AGE
51

HOMETOWN
Portland, Maine

MEDICAL SITUATION
After struggling with ulcerative colitis in the midst of a demanding career as an extreme ski and adventure filmmaker, Brian needed to have an ileostomy.

"To ever think that we are dominating the mountain is foolhardy. The mountain has existed and will exist longer than we ever will. And certainly the mountain has no vested interest in us."

—Brian Sisselman, cinematographer

If someone were to make a movie about Brian Sisselman's life, the film might open with an aerial shot of Pittsfield, Massachusetts, circa mid-1950s. The panorama might include a long shot of snow-draped mountains, with the lens lingering on a small slope called Bousquets. The camera would then capture a dark-haired three-year old boy, sliding down a novice slope on shiny new skis.

A close-up of the child's face would reveal brown eyes lit by an inner fire. The boy seems to belong on the snow. At the bottom of the hill he slows, points his skis inward, then glides to a stop, agile and steady, even at the age of three.

The young boy gazes at a distant mountain—sizeable to competent skiers; colossal to this toddler—and the camera follows his gaze. Wiping melting snowflakes off his long eyelashes, he shades his eyes to capture the sight of skiers gliding down the far-off slopes like birds in flight. The boy's brow furrows momentarily before his small face breaks into a broad grin. Plunging his tiny poles into the snow, he pushes off toward the rope tow to do it all over again.

Cut to a crowded middle school auditorium. It's nighttime, and there's a performance about to begin. People are talking and laughing, kids dart in and out; men, women, and children of all ages congregate, milling about, waiting. The auditorium lights flash and someone yells, "It's time! Take your seats! The movie's about to start!" Still chattering, people migrate to their chairs. The sounds of jackets rustling, chairs scraping the floor, and mothers shushing their children slowly quiets the auditorium as it darkens and a 16-mm movie projector begins its noisy hum.

The camera focuses on the boy, now eight, perched between his parents on a folding chair in the crowded room. Music from the film comes up. The boy's eyes are riveted to the screen in anticipation. Even before the voice on the projector can say the familiar words, "Hi, I'm Warren Miller," the crowd erupts into frenzied hoots and applause. The room is electric with the energy and excitement of a rock concert.

The scene moves to a close-up shot of the boy. Light from the movie projector flickers on his face. People around him blur into the shadows. It's just the boy, the skiers on the screen and the voice from the projector.

A Day of Reckoning

Brian Sisselman—the three-year-old on the slopes,

the schoolboy in the auditorium—might have grown up to become an Olympian, a racer, a jumper, a freestyler, a title holder, or a champion. Instead, he became a filmmaker who has made films about . . . skiing.

It's a variation of the old adage, Those who can't, teach. In this case, it's Those who can't, make movies. Brian does admit to a day of reckoning when his dream of competing in the Olympics were brought to earth with the realization that being a great high school ski racer doesn't necessarily equate to an Olympic athlete. Brian had wowed the locals while growing up, winning local and regional ski races not only in Millbrook School, but at the University of Vermont, as well. Speed and talent notwithstanding, however, Brian couldn't quite measure up against national-level skiers.

Academics and skiing swapped places and Brian began to focus more intently on his studies. During his final year of college, he made a decision that, as it turned out, was pivotal, though at the time he didn't know how important it would be. He was selecting his course work and needed a fine arts class. Scanning the choices in the schedule, his eyes landed on a film class. Why not? He took the course, liked it—and was hooked. Though the fire in his soul for skiing still burned, a new fire was lit that blazes vividly to this day.

Stumbling onto filmmaking during his senior year in college opened up a whole new world to Brian, yet here he was, at the end—not the beginning—of his college career. He had fallen in love with cinematography, but he knew next to nothing about it. Brian knew he had a lot to learn and a long way to go before he could feel competent, let alone adept, at making films, so he made another pivotal decision. Brian applied to and was accepted at UCLA film school.

EXTERIOR SHOT: UCLA DORM PARKING LOT (SUMMER,1975)

Brian is standing beside a Ford Pinto. With him is one of his former professors. The car is packed and overflowing. Brian has just graduated from UCLA Film School.

PROFESSOR: Hey, Brian, before you head back east, why don't you stop off in Hermosa Beach and talk to a guy named Warren Miller? Maybe show him your thesis film.

BRIAN: Warren Miller. Whoa. Now that's a name I haven't heard for years.

PROFESSOR: He's still around. Still makes ski movies. Right up your alley.

BRIAN: Warren Miller. Gee, why not?

Brian still remembers how he felt the day he walked into Warren Miller's office that Friday afternoon in June. He was instantly transported to his boyhood, sitting in auditoriums or museums on crisp fall evenings with scores of other ski aficionados, participating in the annual rite of passage from fall into winter. If you're a skier, then you know that ski season doesn't officially begin until you've watched the latest Warren Miller ski film.

Brian speaks reverently of "the man behind the voice," as if he is still in awe of what happened that day. He was meeting one of the great icons of skiing, truly a living legend. "His world-renowned voice was actually conversing with me. It was the voice behind the magic of the movies, the incarnation of all my boyhood dreams."

It's hard to picture Brian Sisselman uttering these words. Now fifty-one and looking for all the world like the respectable corporate type he is, with cropped and curly salt-and-pepper hair, Brian has a couple of kids of his own waiting for him at home. Yet here he sits in his office in Portland, Maine, sipping coffee and talking about dreams and fantasies and boyhood idols and the time he first met Warren Miller at the ski cinematographer's office in Southern California.

After following Warren into the screening room, Brian sat while the ski maestro threaded up Brian's graduate thesis film, "Ski America." While they viewed the film, Brian became acutely conscious of all the mistakes he'd failed to notice during the editing process. He wished he could sink into his chair, slide to the floor, and slither out the door. If he had, though, he would have missed Warren Miller's "critique" as the credits rolled.

"First, he accused me of stealing his ideas," Brian recalls, "but then he said the film wasn't bad. But then I was really taken when he asked, 'Do you think you might like working in a place like this? Why don't you give me a call on Monday, and we'll talk again.' "

That was a Friday. Monday morning, Brian was back in his office, and Warren Miller spoke the words that would catapult Brian into a career he considers "the ultimate ski bum fantasy"—*Can you start today?*

"That was the beginning of a long history of making ski films," says Brian, who not only began working for Warren Miller the following Monday, but he continued his association with Warren Miller Productions for the next twenty-five years. "I knew the stars had lined up for me. I was at the right place at the right time with the right film in my hand. It was like a dream, and the dream hasn't stopped."

Brian's dream career took him to places that can only be described as extreme. He has literally crossed the globe and back ("I've skied all seven continents," he says), filming the superstars of winter: snowboarders, freestyle skiers, mogul skiers, racers, jumpers, and speed skiers. All of these Brian has captured on film as they skied steep descents and carved fresh tracks through virgin terrain, performing aerials off rocky ledges—sometimes landing, sometimes careening, always (somehow) emerging triumphant. He filmed extreme skiers dropping from helicopters and attacking fifty-degree couloirs before carving up waist-deep powder in the trees.

Watching these ski gods and goddesses soar in logic-defying aerobatics, flouting the laws of physics and treating with utter contempt the gravitational laws by which most of us live, it's easy to forget the man behind the lens. Yet for each rocky ledge from which a snowboarder launched into space or for every glacier an extreme skier descended, there was a cameraman nearby, precariously perched on an adjacent ridge, bearing the weight not only of his own ski gear but of thousands of dollars of filming equipment as well.

If it sounds treacherous, it is. Nevertheless, in spite of the inherently risky nature of this business, the name of the game is safety. "The fewer people we bring out, the better," Brian says. "You don't want to put that many people in extreme environments. I usually go out with myself and three skiers." Depending on where a particular shot will take place, Brian and his crew of skiers will either hike to the location, occasionally roping in together, or fly in by helicopter. "Heli-skiing is an amazing tool for gaining access to impossible spots," he explains. "The helicopter can toe-in while the crew jumps out on the ridge. You're literally straddling the mountain, and when you begin your descent, it's almost like standing next to a wall, with your shoulder brushing the side of the mountain. That's how steep it is."

Of course, getting to those slopes is only half the risk. In remote conditions such as these, the wintertime weather can change unexpectedly and dramatically. "Sometimes we're shooting hours from civilization in an extreme location that has no mercy for anyone. If you're an hour away from camp and bad weather comes in, you run the risk of not being able to find your way back."

Then there's the ever-present peril of avalanches. "No school can tell you how to survive an avalanche. If you get caught in one, it's just bad luck. Once I was filming five of the best skiers in the world in Canada. I remember at one point telling the crew, because the light was bad, 'Let's stop now and go back down for some lunch.' While we were down the mountain, we heard about a massive avalanche that killed nine guests from our lodge. They had been in the same area that we had been filming."

It goes without saying that in an outdoor business like Brian's, which requires a hearty dose of both artistic vision and physical stamina, good health is a prerequisite. And for many years, good health was a given for Brian. He claims, in fact, that he never had any physical problems growing up. That all changed dramatically when Brian turned thirty-one years old.

"I was living in Colorado at the time," Brian recalls. "I was married to Jenna by then, and I began to get bouts of severe diarrhea that would strike randomly and without notice. I couldn't figure out what was causing it. There was no connection between what I ate and when I would have these attacks."

Brian told nobody about these episodes, even when they began to interfere with his work. "One time while filming I knew I was going to have to leave immediately," he recalls. "I made some sort of an excuse—like a piece of camera equipment broke—and I raced down the mountain to find a toilet. It was definitely getting to be a problem."

The defining moment came while filming in the backcountry of Colorado. Brian, who by then had lost a significant amount of weight, knew that the situation was out of control. He checked himself into the hospital, and for the first time in his life heard the term "ulcerative colitis." The doctor examining him even mentioned the possibility of surgery.

Brian remembers being overwhelmed with disbelief when he heard the news. "I'd had no warm up," he says. "I was angry and determined that this was not going to happen to me." At that point, he says, he went into serious denial. He began Prednisone treatments, which helped get the symptoms under control—so much so that he assumed he was a cured man. He convinced himself that none of this was happening to him.

For nearly two years he fooled himself into believing he was well. When his symptoms returned, he pretended to be already booked when freelance assignments came up, rather than admit he was too sick to take the job. Like a man stranded on the side of a mountain, bracing himself against the avalanche that would rip him from his perch and send him plummeting into a heap below, Brian felt desperate, despondent, and vulnerable. Only then did he begin to consider surgery.

Making the decision to have the surgery was overwhelming for Brian. The thought of changing his body so dramatically did not seem like a good choice. He would also be giving up the hope that the medication would permanently control his disease. Brian and Jenna recall sitting at their home in Vail, Colorado, knowing their world had been invaded by this uncontrollable disease. Going over the options—or lack of options—they knew that the surgical route would be frightening and final. Brian would need a lot of luck to continue his filming career.

With great reluctance, Brian submitted to ostomy surgery. Recovery was slow and painful—physically ("I guess I have a low pain threshold," he confesses) and emotionally ("It was overwhelming to deal with the changes."). There was also the dramatic change in self-image.

"I think what happened scared him," Jenna says. In the beginning, she was the one who changed Brian's bags for him. Her early attempts were awkward. "The first time took two hours!" she recalls, shaking her head. In his early funk, Brian remembers telling his wife, "Honey, you're going to have to help me with this for the rest of my life!"

But, as Brian says now, eventually human nature takes over. "You take one step, then the next, and slowly you get better." It wasn't long before he began to manage the pouch himself, a task he can now accomplish in three to seven minutes. He spent the summer recuperating, taking walks, and sitting in the sunshine. By August, he felt good enough to accept a job filming in the Colorado Sand Dunes, with surgical tubes still hanging out of his stomach. The following winter, Brian found himself in a Twin Otter seaplane, skimming over the waves of Drake Passage, en route to perhaps the most dangerous filming expedition of his career: Antarctica, one of the most hostile and desolate regions in the world.

He felt great.

He was back where he belonged.

The dream was alive.

Stopping all medications and opting for surgery has proven to be one of the best decisions of Brian's life. He continues making films around the world and is currently producing a natural history show for television appropriately called "Adventure Crusoe."

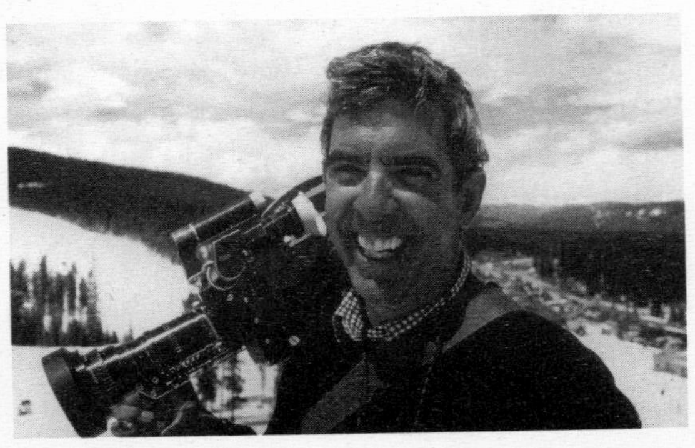

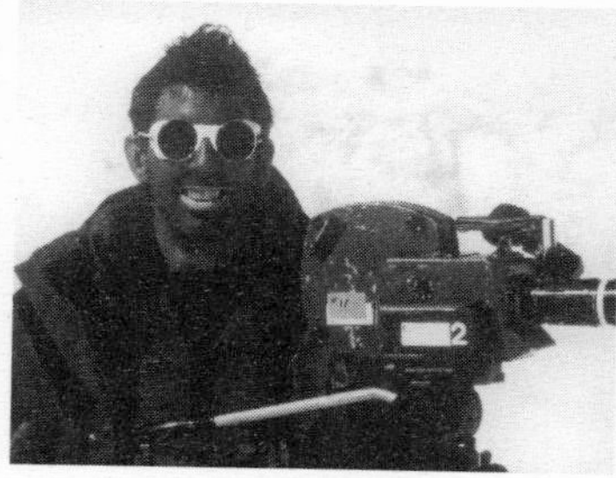

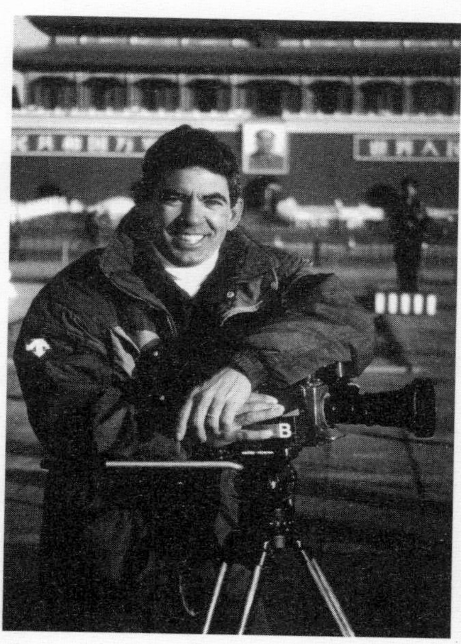

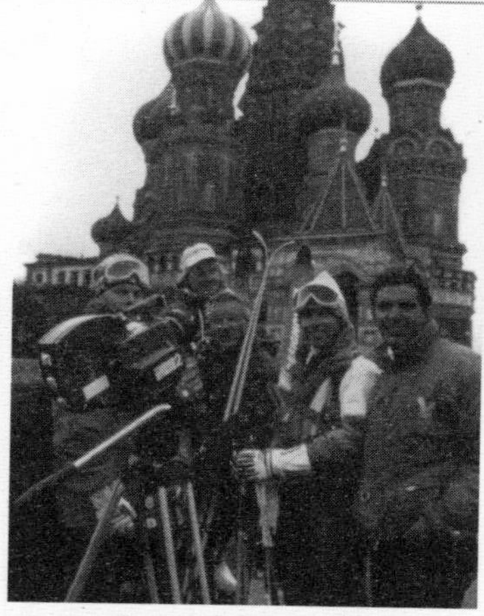

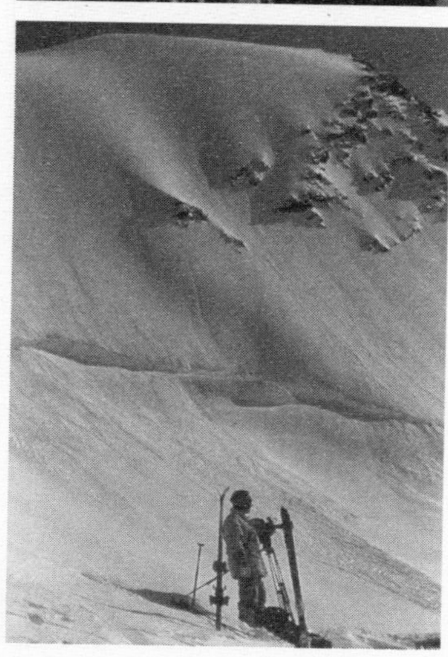

"Have camera will travel" was the way Brian Sisselman lived for years as a veteran director and cameraman for Warren Miller Films. Brian has traveled the world and filmed on all seven continents, including exotic locales such as China, Antarctica, and Russia.

Despite the often harsh conditions, Brian says his ostomy has never stopped him from doing his job, whether it's filming skiers at 18,000 feet in the Himalayas of India, or being dropped from a helicopter on some rugged mountain peak miles away from civilization in Greenland.

For Better or for Worse

WAYNE PLISS

AGE

41

HOMETOWN

Largo, Florida

MEDICAL SITUATION

After developing ulcerative colitis in his late twenties, he endured the disease for twelve years before having an ileostomy six days before his wedding.

Not too many guys spend their wedding night in a hospital bed with a fever spiking at 105 and a bride dozing in a cot three feet away. But that's what happened to Wayne Pliss on a sultry June night just six days after ileostomy surgery removed both his large intestine and his rectum. Contrary to the advice of his surgeon, Wayne and Connie Pliss decided to keep their date with the preacher, in spite of the interference that major abdominal surgery represented. Wayne calls it a blip on the radar screen of life.

So why didn't Wayne simply postpone the wedding until he had fully recovered? "All the friends and relatives were already on their way," says Wayne matter-of-factly. "Connie's parents had reserved their country club for the reception. Why change things at the last minute?"

Why, indeed? After all, how much trouble could it be, really, to arrive at the church in an ambulance rather than a limousine, roll down the aisle in a wheelchair, and take a one-minute shuffle around the dance floor instead of a ballroom whirl?

"I mean, come *awn*!" says Wayne, and that's how he talks—like someone who's lived half his life on the streets of New York. Born in Queens and raised on Long Island, Wayne is as accustomed to the crowds and congestion of New York City as his wife Connie is to the rural quiet of Dowagiac, Michigan, a city of 8,000 "where you can get anywhere in five minutes and the Main Street has only two stoplights." And Wayne isn't one to second-guess himself. "When we made the decision to have the surgery, all the wedding plans were set, so we decided to go ahead with it," he says. "I don't know what the fuss is all about."

The "fuss" Wayne is referring to might have something to do with an ABC news crew dropping in unexpectedly on the Pliss wedding. Evidently getting wind of the event from the ambulance company that Connie hired to transport Wayne from the hospital to the church, the news team stuck around long enough to film Wayne and Connie making their wedding vows and to interview Wayne on a stretcher afterward. Later that night back at the hospital, the newlyweds watched the two-minute blurb where Wayne, looking, in his words, "like a concentration camp survivor," lay in agony. He had a deep incision bisecting his abdomen, an ileostomy pouch awkwardly affixed to his side, and his state of awareness distorted by the constant flow of morphine into his veins.

In spite of the physical inconveniences, Wayne and Connie did manage a little conjugal romp that first night together. Okay, so perhaps he did regret it later, as giggling nurses tended to his ruptured sutures. But you didn't find him second-guessing himself, either. "We have a very active sex life," he remarks with only a hint of modesty.

A Little Background

Connie Pliss is no stranger to hospitals—or to bowel disorders. Her first husband suffered from Crohn's disease, and she and Wayne actually met as a result of the loss of Wayne's first wife, Kathy, who had died in November 1989 just four months after being diagnosed with colon cancer. Connie, who relocated to Florida with her family when she was in her early twenties, was an oncology social worker at Morton Plant Hospital in Florida when she was assigned to Kathy Pliss' case. Connie remembers being struck by how stunningly gorgeous Kathy was with long, beautiful blonde hair. "It's always a difficult thing when someone that young comes in to die," muses Connie, a striking blonde herself.

It was Connie who put Wayne in touch with grievance counselors after Kathy passed away. She didn't think about him until three months later when he contacted her, still devastated by his loss. "When Kathy was diagnosed," Wayne explains, "everyone told me she was dying. Even my doctor pulled me aside one day and said he'd gladly take a miracle, but other than a miracle, she has no chance. I refused to believe it. I even dragged her to a clinic in the Bahamas that specializes in alternative cancer treatments." It was, he says, the worst three weeks in his life. The aggressive therapy didn't help and Wayne, seeing Kathy deteriorate, finally brought her back to Florida and admitted her into a hospital. "By then, the cancer had spread like wildfire, and she didn't want to fight it anymore," he says. "She died a week later."

Wayne took the loss hard. He tells of being unable to sleep, suffering from frequent nightmares in which he'd wake up drenched in sweat. He had trouble facing people, and he became more and more isolated. He'd spend hours simply walking on the beach. In desperation, he called Connie, the only person he remembered from his days at the hospital. Restricted by hospital rules that forbade her from providing counseling to non-patients, Connie referred Wayne to a hospice worker who had set up a private practice. Through intensive counseling, Wayne finally turned the corner in his grieving.

A few months later he contacted Connie again. This time, the call was personal—he asked her out to lunch. But Connie hesitated, having just come out of a difficult marriage and raising two young sons alone. "I knew it took a lot of courage for him to ask me out, so I agreed to meet for lunch," said Connie, who wanted to be sensitive to what Wayne was going through. As one lunch date led to another, Connie became concerned about getting involved with someone so newly bereaved and whether Wayne would be a good influence on the boys. Taking things slowly, the two developed a relationship that eventually began to deepen because of their differences ("She never knew what a football was until I met her!" he says) and their accord ("When he tried to have a good relationship with my boys, I knew he was someone I could trust," she says).

The Roots of the Disease

Though Connie was aware at the time she and Wayne were dating that he had ulcerative colitis, she didn't realize how serious things were—possibly because he preferred it that way and kept his complaints to a minimum. Wayne's health problems began in his high school years. A particularly severe bout was serious enough to alarm his parents and compel them to take Wayne to a specialist in Manhattan. By the time the physician examined Wayne, however, the symptoms had dissipated and the doctor pronounced him "fine." Wayne was advised to watch his diet and "steer clear" of roughage.

It wasn't until Wayne was twenty-eight, after becoming seriously ill with abdominal cramps, bleeding, and loose stools, that his family physician officially diagnosed him with ulcerative colitis. Right about that time, he began to experience the kind of symptoms that any young, single guy would dread. "I remember one time I was on a double date with a friend of mine from Miami," says Wayne, now a muscular forty-one-year-old businessman from Clearwater, Florida, who stays in shape by competing in marathons and triathlons in his spare time. "We went out to a restaurant in Tampa. I think we had Italian food. We were driving home and were about ten minutes away from my condo, and I couldn't make it. I had a loose, messy bowel movement, right there in the car."

There were other dating disasters. "Connie and I were on our way to a jazz concert," he recalls, "and I soiled my pants in the car. I was humiliated, but Connie handled it great. We went back to her house where I showered and cleaned up." Connie remembers another episode that occurred when she and Wayne were dining in a nice restaurant. Wayne had on white slacks at the time, which only amplified the disaster. "It really didn't bother me," she remembers. "I just felt bad for him."

Wayne tells of a time when he couldn't even make the half-hour drive from Connie's house to his condo without having an accident. "I got so fed up with losing bowel control that I'd toss my dirty shorts into the garbage can by the pool rather than deal with the mess."

But by then, Connie was totally committed in the relationship. It never occurred to her, even as Wayne's health deteriorated and her role in the relationship shifted from girlfriend to caregiver, to withdraw from him or tell him to check back in a year when he was better. Even as their wedding date approached and Wayne was so ill that he needed to lean against a wall for support, all she cared about was getting him better. "It got so bad that Wayne began sleeping on the couch at my place," says Connie, "because he couldn't make the drive home. I finally said, 'Enough. This can't go on. You've got to go to the hospital.' "

To Wayne, checking himself into a hospital was tantamount to admitting that he was going to die. He'd seen it happen once already with his first wife. Connie, however, knew that if Wayne didn't get treatment immediately he would die. So she took him to the emergency room. To her dismay he "checked out okay" and was told to go home and eat a bland, liquid diet. "But that's what he's been doing!" contended Connie, who pointed out that Wayne wasn't even keeping water down, let alone the bland foods she'd been preparing for him.

Stubbornly, she refused to budge. A specialist was contacted, and Wayne was finally admitted for hospitalization and more tests. "When I think about how it might have been if we'd simply complied with this ER doctor and gone home I cringe. Wayne would probably be dead," Connie fumes. "Think of all the people who are afraid to challenge or question their doctors, or who have limited English. That's frustrating."

In the hospital, Wayne received massive doses of steroids to reduce his inflammation and frequent injections of pain medication. According to Connie, he ended up with a fist-sized decubitus ulcer on his hip, which remains to this day, the result of a subcutaneous infection from frequent injections in the same spot. Drug treatment, however, was ineffective, and it gradually became evident that surgery would be necessary.

For Wayne's parents, the thought of their son wearing an ostomy pouch was difficult, and there was a brief flurry of activity as they insisted he explore other alternatives. They discussed antidepressants and even toyed with the idea of transferring Wayne to the renowned Cleveland Clinic. Wayne was so sick, however, that after weighing the pros and cons and praying about it at great length with Connie, everyone agreed that surgery was the only option. Although he had no fear going in because of his deep faith in God, emerging from the anesthesia was a different story.

"I was scared," he recalls, "because I was in so much pain. I hadn't anticipated that and must have pressed the morphine button three hundred times that first hour. Trying to get up was brutal and blowing the blow bottles to try to expand my lungs was pure torture. As if my physical pain wasn't enough, I remember lifting up my hospital gown to check out my incision and nearly getting sick at the sight." To make matters worse Wayne began to hallucinate from the morphine, thinking at times he was hanging upside down or that the flowers in his room were actually menacing creatures. He kept spiking fevers and also needed several blood transfusions. He was a mess!

While Wayne was battling one post-operative complication after another, the clock kept ticking and the calendar date kept moving closer and closer to the date Wayne and Connie had set for their wedding. Wayne's doctor was concerned and insisted they either reschedule the wedding or have it in the hospital chapel. Wayne wouldn't budge and insisted they leave the date and proceed with their plans. The two went round and round on the subject until Wayne eventually prevailed, but not without agreeing to sign a waiver, releasing the hospital of liability.

The Physical Side

Like any new bride, Connie was looking forward to the intimacy from which she and Wayne had abstained during their courtship. The fact that the groom was fifty pounds underweight and "looked ghastly—like a skeleton" did nothing to lessen her anticipation. She did panic slightly, she admits, when a day or two after his surgery, she caught a glimpse of his behind ("Those hospital gowns are indecent!") as he shuffled up and down the hospital hallway. "His buttocks were perfectly round," she recalls, laughing. "There was no crack! But the nurse reassured me that Wayne's rear end was just swollen and puffy and that it would return to normal."

Six days later, on June 15th at 2:00 in the afternoon at Lakeside Community Chapel, a gathering of about ninety people witnessed the union of Wayne and Connie Pliss—right on schedule. The bride wore a tailored, long-sleeved gown of ivory lace, her soft blonde curls crowned with a garland of baby's breath and peach-colored roses. Looking gaunt and pale, but spruced up with a fresh haircut and a shave, the groom wore a navy suit with a rose tucked neatly in his lapel. As she and Wayne stood before the altar and repeated their vows, Connie had to stifle a giggle when Pastor Steve Kreloff came to the portion of the vow in which he asked if Connie would take Wayne to be her lawfully wedded husband, for better or for worse. How much worse can it get? she remembers thinking.

Connie and Wayne's wedding night wasn't the stuff dreams are made of. She still remembers wandering the hospital hallway at 11:00 p.m. in her wedding gown, waiting for her brother to bring her street clothes. "Despite the strangeness of the circumstances, I was happy," says Connie. "We had been through so much, and now we had hope again. I felt like a huge weight had been lifted."

A week later, she and Wayne were permitted to leave the hospital after signing another waiver and spend their official honeymoon at a local resort in St. Petersburg. Much of her time was spent changing dressings, tending to the infection on Wayne's hip, and helping with the ostomy appliance. She even nursed his severely blistered sunburn, the result of a bad combination of residual steroids and too much sun. But despite these physical nuisances—any one of which would have dampened the ardor of most couples—the newlyweds were undaunted. "We enjoyed our physical intimacy so much," Connie confesses, "and we felt so happy to be together with so much to look forward to."

And the ostomy? Now approaching their eleventh wedding anniversary, both Connie and Wayne insist it's never been an issue, and nor was the ostomy a hindrance on having children. Wayne and Connie have two sons of their own about to enter grade school and kindergarten.

As for their physical relationship, "I wear a one-piece pouch," Wayne explains, "and when we make love, I just tape it up. For us," he adds, chuckling, "it's not the pouch that's a problem—it's our two little boys being able to hear us!"

Looking back, Connie thinks she was well prepared for Wayne's ostomy from her time in the medical profession. "As a new bride," she says, "I wasn't turned off or offended. And now, I never even think about it when we're together. I'm just so glad to have him alive and healthy." In their ten years together, only once did the pouch leak during sexual intimacy. "We just laughed and jumped in the shower," Connie says. "We laugh about everything."

And it is with that laughter, faith, and a mutual commitment to stick it out that has seen Wayne and Connie through sickness and health, and enabled them to "love, honor and cherish each other . . . for better and for worse."

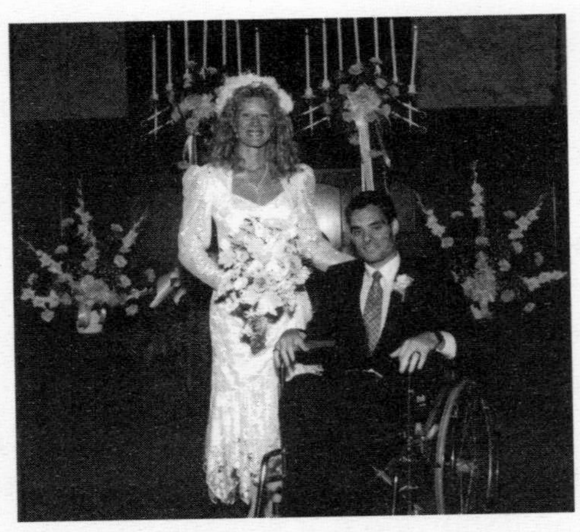

For Wayne Pliss, nothing comes between him and his woman . . . especially ileostomy surgery. Just six days after surgeons removed his colon and rectum, Wayne made it to the altar on time to marry his wife, Connie.

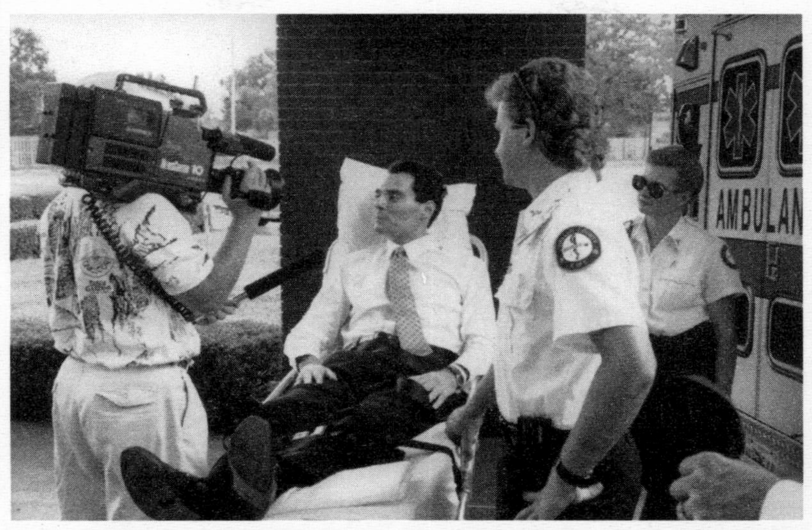

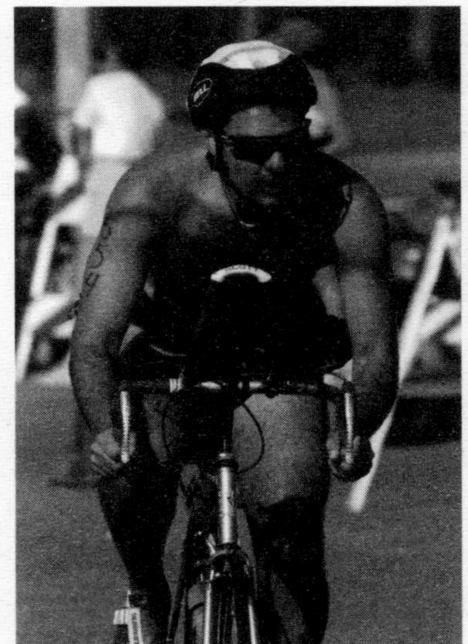

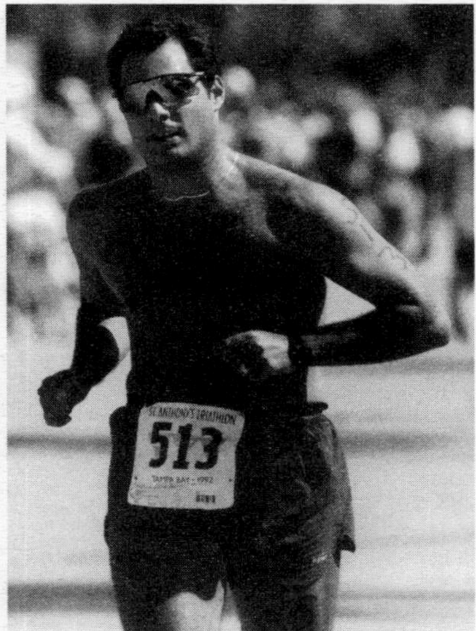

The notoriety of getting married so soon after surgery brought out the local TV camera crews to capture the event. Today, Wayne is active in business but still finds time to compete in endurance events such as 10k races and triathlons, and he loves to speak to anyone about the benefits of ostomy surgery.

Feeling Singularly Blessed

PAULA ERWIN-TOTH

AGE
46

HOMETOWN
Deerfield, Ohio

MEDICAL SITUATION
Born with a congenital birth defects—bladder exstrophy (when the bladder is outside the body) and bilateral hip dysplasia (dislocated hips)—Paula experienced numerous surgeries, including a urostomy (ileal conduit) at the age of ten.

Her earliest memories are of hospitals.

One of them happened when she looked down and saw a body cast stretching from her underarms to her ankles. This wasn't a very large body cast, mind you. She was, after all, only two-years-old.

Another time, she was gazing from the fourth floor of her hospital room at her two older brothers—one holding her pet cat—and her father on the sidewalk below, waving. Brave little girl that she was, she waved back. But she also cried.

Finally, there was the time when she was being packed in ice and lying very still, eyes fixed on the ceiling, as nurses bustled in and out. What else was there for a feverish child to do but mathematically divide the holes in the ceiling tiles into a logical grid?

Paula Erwin-Toth knows hospitals. She knows them not only because the first ten years of her life were spent in and out of them, but also because now, as an adult, she has devoted nearly every waking hour to caring for people who are facing the kind of surgery she herself experienced when she was ten. Currently the Director of Enterostomal Therapy Nursing at the renowned Cleveland Clinic in Ohio, Paula is a woman on a mission. For her, ET nursing is more than a job; it's a way of giving back. Giving back on a personal level, but also in a broader, grander sense, making a difference in the still-emerging field of medicine in which she specializes.

The story of Paula's remarkable life begins with birth defects and deformity but has been enriched by good timing, fortuitous locale, and an indomitable spirit. It's a story of heroes in basements, a close-knit and supportive family, and a mother who somehow grasped the difference between concern and solicitousness. It's a story of an exceptional child, whose experiences, though far from typical, neither squelched nor stymied the enthusiasm and exhilaration characteristic of most children. It's a tale of understated courage, quiet determination, and, in the end, quintessential childhood.

Here, in her words, is her story.

I was born on a July morning in 1955 in Akron, Ohio. Those were the days when expectant mothers were whisked away to the delivery room while the dads cooled their heels in the waiting room. Unfortunately for my dad, he had to cool his heels several hours longer than usual after I was born. All he knew—all he was told—was that there was "a problem" with the baby. Four hours later, he sat in the driver's seat of his car, heading down the block to take me to Children's Hospital. Perched beside him in the front seat was a student nurse, clutching me—five hours old and newly christened Paula Lyn Erwin—in her arms.

Back in the maternity ward, my mother, dispossessed of her third child and only daughter, demanded an explanation. At this point, no one knew what was wrong, only that the prognosis didn't look good. One well-meaning but misinformed doctor urged my mother to steel herself to the fact that if I lived, I would probably never walk, would most likely be deaf and retarded, and would certainly be incontinent of both urine and stool. Perhaps the kindest thing they could do as parents, this doctor tentatively suggested, would be to not feed me and let me die. Fortunately my mom, who had been an X-ray technician before settling down to raise a family, possessed just enough medical background and a fierce maternal instinct to promptly dismiss the outlandish suggestion. For her, the thing to do was to find out what was wrong and go from there.

The technical term for what was wrong with me is congenital exstrophy of the bladder and bilateral hip dysplasia. Basically what this means is that, because my abdominal wall didn't close, my bladder was inside out and upside down outside my body, and both my hips were dislocated. This rare congenital condition occurs approximately once in every 60,000 live births.

My first major surgery to rebuild my pelvis and close the bladder wall took place when I was six months old. Two more surgeries followed, one when I was eight months and another at two-and-a-half years of age. The last one required a full body cast, known as a hip spica cast, to set the bones in my pelvis. Early on, there was some doubt about whether I'd ever be able to walk. To the surprise of the doctor who had grimly told my mother it would never happen, I did finally walk at age four.

Mom turned to me and said, "Paula, come here," and I came. When the doctor heard that I walked, he apologized and said, "Then again, I could be wrong."

Besides the hip surgeries, there were bladder problems. Because my bladder was so small, the urine couldn't run out fast enough. Consequently, urine backed up into my kidneys and caused, among other things, kidney stones. The stones had to be surgically removed through large, painful flank incisions. By the time I turned ten, I'd had six of those brutal surgeries. You can imagine the scars I have on my back. I remember once wearing a two-piece bathing suit as a teenager when a stranger actually came up to me and asked about the scars. Feeling impish, I said, "You know those magic acts where they cut people in half? They don't always work." I think he believed me!

The doctors who predicted I'd be incontinent of both urine and stool were only partly correct. I did have bowel control, but a lack of urinary sphincters, combined with a very short urethra, precluded my ability to hold or control urine flow. The only way to manage incontinence, of course, is by wearing protective clothing. I'm talking about diapers. Back in the good old days, before Pampers and Huggies and those wonderfully convenient adhesive closures, mothers diapered their babies in cloth and secured the diaper with safety pins. The diapers were then covered with plastic panties, ringed at the waist and thigh openings with elastic. Wet or soiled diapers weren't tossed in the landfills the way they are today. They were washed and dried, along with the rest of the laundry.

Luckily for both mothers and babies, diaper-wearing days are limited. Eventually children get potty-trained and those diaper-wearing, diaper-washing days fade blissfully into a vague and distant memory.

Not so for me. I wore diapers all the time. That's "all" as in every day, every night. I wore them as a toddler, when it wasn't that unusual to still be in diapers. I wore them as little girl, when all my friends had graduated into "big girl" panties. I wore them going into kindergarten for the first time, and I wore them all through public elementary school when my "differentness" could be ignored no longer.

There weren't special schools for kids like me. I was mainstreamed before the term became fashionable, and I endured the jabs and the jokes that come with the territory. You can say all you like about how wonderful children are, but don't forget that kids can be mean. In my memory, girls were worse than boys: they would giggle and point and gossip and whisper. When I was in the first grade, for example, one of my classmates told everyone that I wore diapers. And though some of my teachers were sympathetic, not all of them understood. One teacher, in fact, told me plainly that I was lazy, and that if I had some discipline, I wouldn't have to wear diapers anymore.

Like any child, the older I got, the more responsible I was for my own toilet routine. The fact that I was incontinent and that my routine was a little different from other kids' didn't matter. It was mostly a question of doing what had to be done and doing it as discreetly as possible. I carried extra diapers with me to school and stored them in a locker or in the teachers' lounge. Since I had no bladder control, I didn't have a choice about when my diaper would be wet or dry. If the diaper was wet, it was up to me to take care of it. This, of course, wasn't always convenient. I remember once being on the playground, trying to determine how wet the diaper was and whether I could go down the slide and not leave a streak before having to change. When I finally did have to change my diaper, I'd go to the teachers' restroom, then wrap up the wet one in a plastic bag and carry it home. Walking home was another story. Try walking home from school in an Ohio winter wearing wet diapers. Winters were the worst. I was always cold.

I suppose it's easy to look back and wonder how a mother could allow her child to go to school wearing diapers, knowing full well that she'd be teased or taunted or laughed at or ostracized. My mother didn't have a choice. For my family, as bad as my health problems were, they paled when compared to another health crisis we faced. Shortly after I was born, my father was diagnosed with paranoid schizophrenia. For many years Dad was in and out of the VA Psychiatric Hospital.

In order to provide for the family, Mom had to work. My brothers and I became forerunners of what would later be termed "latchkey kids." We fixed dinner, did our homework, and cleaned up the house before Mom got home. And even when Dad was around, we helped out and didn't complain. I don't remember whining much as a kid. I think I must have intuitively sensed that Mom's problems were more important than mine.

That's not to say Mom wasn't my advocate. She was extremely protective of me, and she was relentless in trying to find out what was wrong and how to help. She was the one who arranged for special bathroom privileges for me at school. Normally she's shy and quiet, but when it came to getting medical information, she was indefatigable. One time, during an office visit in which Mom pummeled a doctor with questions, he said to her, "I see you've been reading again."

"Yes, and I'd like an answer," she replied. On the other hand, Mom also knew that as I grew older, she had to give me some space. I remember my aunts marveling once at how Mom watched me swinging from a tree and dropping into a lake. When they asked how she could remain so calm, Mom responded, "I don't want to turn her into an invalid." Then she expressed what probably sums up her entire approach to raising me: "If Paula didn't have these health problems, would what she's doing bother me?"

I think Mom's outlook probably explains why, in spite of everything I went through, I was really not so different from other kids. I was a cheerleader in junior high school. I liked to run and play soccer. I shot a mean free throw and could hold my own playing one-on-one basketball with my brother. I loved to swim. And I broke my femur once playing football with my brothers and the neighborhood boys. The frequent surgeries were merely the backdrop. In between hospitalizations, life went on.

Right about the time I turned ten, the decision was made to perform an ileal conduit, or what's commonly known as a urinary diversion. My doctors felt this procedure would be the only way to deal once and for all with my incessant kidney infections, kidney stones, and hemorrhages. The year was 1965, and at the time, this kind of pediatric surgery was just being pioneered in the Akron area. No one explained to me at first what was going on. I remember everyone crying around me—my family, my friends, even my urologist—but they didn't tell me why. I was sure they were crying because they knew that I was dying, and I was terrified. At last my surgeon, Dr. William Sharp, came in and carefully explained the procedure. He even drew a picture that showed where the ostomy would go. I looked at him and asked point blank, "You mean I'm not dying?"

"Heck no, you're not dying!" he exclaimed. I felt so relieved!

My surgery date conflicted with the Soap Box Derby in Akron. This was a big deal. Kids came from all over the world to participate. There was a big parade featuring movie stars and celebrities. Many of the stars would then visit the kids at Children's Hospital. The day my urinary diversion was performed, my visitors included Frankie Avalon, Fess Parker, and "some guy named Glenn Ford" as I told my mother later. I remember Mr. Ford placing a cool cloth on my head. I must have looked like death warmed over, but it felt nice.

Even though my first words when I saw the ostomy were "It looks yucky!", the biggest adjustment was learning how to manage the urine flow. Those were the early days when ostomy appliances were in the Dark Ages. I was given a stoma plate made of latex and metal. The pouch was also made of latex. The only way to get the appliance to stick was to paint latex cement on, wait until the cement was partly dry, and then attach the pouch and secure it with a belt. In order to remove the pouch, a solvent was necessary.

Not only was this method problematic for people with latex sensitivities like me, it also wasn't very efficient. Like a leaky faucet, the urine would saturate the cement around the pouch. I ended up having to change the pouch a couple of times a day, and occasionally having to soak in an oatmeal bath to relieve the discomfort of skin irritations from the solvent. But I had lived all my life in bulky diapers, and I was accustomed to being wet most of the time, so none of this mattered. Just having my urine go into a pouch was like a miracle. Not only that, I could wear panties instead of diapers! Heaven!

My hero in those early days was a woman named Norma Gill, whose work at the Cleveland Clinic with ostomy patients was becoming well known in the Akron area. Though the nurses at Children's Hospital were competent and caring, they were also untrained in stoma management and care. When Norma Gill agreed to see me, it was as if the Lord heard my prayer. The woman who single-handedly pioneered the medical specialty known as Enterostomal Therapy stepped into my hospital room, took charge, and changed my life. She explained, in no uncertain terms, to the nurses as well as the surgeons what needed to be done. She was a lifesaver.

Norma became my personal mentor and friend. I remember going to her house for check-ups, which actually took place in her bedroom, while her two poodles sat at the corner of her bed and watched. Those were the years when the only place to pick up your ostomy supplies was out of Norma's basement. If she knew she wasn't going to be home, she would leave the equipment in her garage.

As Norma worked with "her kids" and saw areas that needed improvement, she communicated those needs to ostomy manufacturers. Gradually the equipment improved, and as the equipment improved, so did my quality of life. It wasn't long before those diaper-wearing, diaper-changing days did—at last—fade blissfully into a vague and distant memory.

Though she entered college intent on studying English, Paula Erwin-Toth switched her major to nursing after unexpectedly losing her eldest brother to leukemia. She earned both her Bachelor's and her Master's degrees in Nursing from the University of Akron. She assumed the role of Director of Enterostomal Therapy Nursing at the Cleveland Clinic in 1990, taking the baton from Norma Gill.

Today, Paula keeps busy seeing patients, educating students, and lecturing in the United States and around the world. In addition to the numerous surgeries she experienced as a child, she has also faced additional surgeries as an adult, including multiple hernia repairs and a hysterectomy to remove an ovarian tumor. Despite these blows, she considers herself "singularly blessed." She lives with her husband, Jim, and their assorted animals in Deerfield, Ohio, and they maintain a close relationship with Jim's daughter, Marya, and their grandson, Vincent.

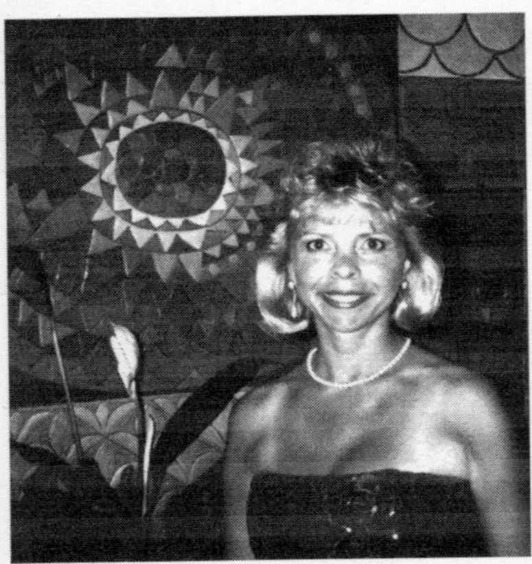

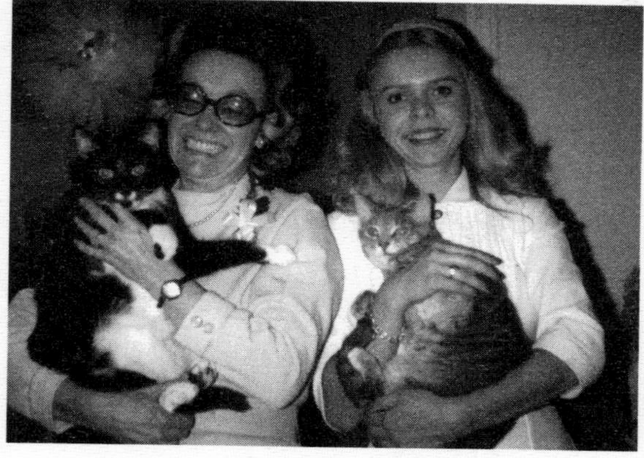

Paula Erwin-Toth got her first bad break the moment she was born. Doctors diagnosed her with two congenital birth defects: hip displasia and bladder exstrophy, where the bladder is formed outside the body.

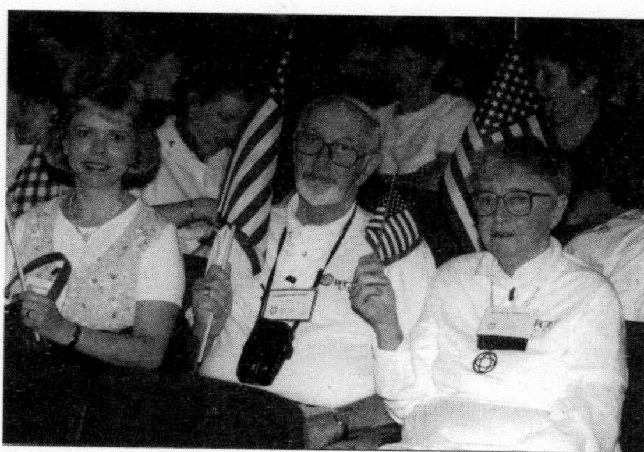

She spent her early childhood years wearing diapers and shuttling in and out of hospitals before undergoing urostomy surgery at the tender age of ten. Paula has never let her medical situation keep her from living a full and exciting life.

Paula married Jim and today is recognized as one of the top ET nurses in the country. She is currently working at the Cleveland Clinic.

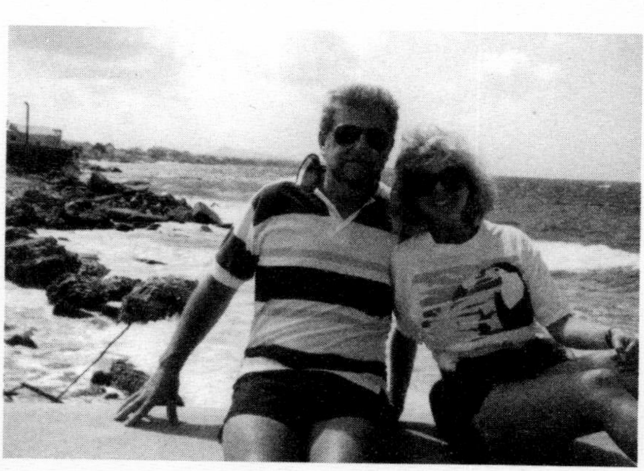

Beyond the Chutes

TONY BELL

AGE
21

HOMETOWN
Harveyville, Kansas

MEDICAL SITUATION
He was born with an imperforate anus, which led to multiple surgeries and a colostomy at the tender age of nine.

It was the final day of a four-day rodeo camp, and seventeen-year-old Tony Bell was psyched. He'd spent many long and painful hours honing his skills on the mechanical bulls and practicing when he could on real animals in the arena. He had learned to adjust his body to the shuffle, twist, and roll of bull riding—so different from the lurch and jar of bronco riding. Call him foolhardy, but Tony discovered that he preferred the solid rocking motion of a Brahman bull to the whiplash created by a bucking horse.

Tony could visualize the nearly two-ton beast he would soon straddle: the dense, slippery hide; the massive shoulders; the powerful flank muscles; the colossal chest; and the deadly horns, or "clown stabbers," as his instructors called them. He could see the wild, almost frenzied stare in the animal's eyes, and he could hear the angry snort from its nostrils as it shook its head trying to gore anything it could find. In his mind, he even heard the shouts and cheers from the stands as he completed his eight-second ride, after which the bullfighter clowns came running out to distract the bull while Tony scrambled out of harm's way.

Tony had been stepped on before, and he could still recall the weight and power of the hooves as they cut deep into his chest. He can still vividly remember how his good buddy, Dan Sears, nearly died after a bull stepped on the back of his head a few years ago. Dan spent six months in a coma after that accident and would never ride again.

None of that mattered just then though. All that mattered was now—this rodeo, this arena, and this bull. The teen bull rider sat behind the chutes, waiting his turn along with the other cowboys preparing for their own chance to ride. For the umpteenth time Tony checked his gear. The heavy bull rope, the slightly tarnished bell, used to annoy the animal so it would buck harder, the thick, well-worn glove with its familiar odor of rosin mixed with leather and bull sweat. He felt for his spurs with his boots, examined his chaps, and nervously adjusted his Stetson. He was ready.

And then, moments before it was time to enter the chute and mount the bull, he bowed his head and whispered the familiar words of the Cowboy Prayer. It had already been prayed earlier that morning when all the cowboys had gathered together before the rodeo began. But Tony uttered it again, this time making it personal.

Heavenly Father, I pause, mindful of the many blessings You have bestowed upon me. I ask that You be with me at this rodeo. And I pray that You guide me, too, in the Arena of Life . . . .

No Fences

Tony Bell had always wanted to be a cowboy. When he was young, watching John Wayne flicks with his dad, he would admire the endless prairies "where everything was wild and free, and there were no fences and you could go wherever you wanted to go." It stirred something deep within him.

Maybe it was in his blood. His father had farmed over 1,500 acres while Tony was growing up. It was the same Kansas land his ancestors had worked way back when. For Tony, now twenty years old, being a cowboy is his way of perpetuating a fading heritage. "People are becoming too modern and not remembering where they came from," he reflects. "I don't want to forget my roots. Farming is who I am. My grandfather passed this farm down to my dad. Someday, it will be mine."

If these words are music to a father's ears, no doubt it's because they represent more than the passing of the torch from father to son. Indeed, Tony's dad, Marvin, has mixed feelings about Tony's dream to become a farmer. "It's a tough way to make a living," he concedes. Yet, he has seen Tony overcome some tremendous obstacles at a very young age and—and become a better man because of it. Tony's first up-and-down challenge came when he was only minutes old.

Early Days

Cindy Bell had resigned herself to the fact that she'd never bear a child, which is why she and her husband decided to adopt their first two children. When their second child was two, however, Cindy began to experience health problems that persisted for weeks.

While most women would recognize the symptoms of early pregnancy—nausea, vomiting, and fatigue—those thoughts never occurred to Cindy. After all, she had never known what it was like to carry a baby and had long since given up any hope of becoming pregnant.

When the symptoms persisted, Cindy made an appointment with her family doctor. Familiar enough with her history not to suspect pregnancy either, Cindy's doctor focused on her gall bladder. He ordered a series of tests, including an upper GI and an X-ray. The tests revealed nothing wrong.

Two weeks later, still feeling ill and intuitively sensing that she might be expecting, Cindy insisted on a pregnancy test. To everyone's amazement, it was discovered that Cindy was almost three months along! She was excited but horrified. What if the X-ray had affected her unborn child? But there was nothing Cindy could do now except to find a more competent physician for her prenatal care. She was furious, but she never told her original doctor—after Tony was born—about her son's congenital birth defect. What was the point? Life had to go on.

Cindy's labor was long, difficult, and ultimately risky, and she ended up needing a Cesarean section. Cindy's husband, Marvin, was in the delivery room when his third child was born. "I remember the doctor lifting the baby up and the sudden silence that filled the room. I got this sense that something was terribly wrong."

The doctor did his best to explain the situation to Mr. Bell, but even he was perplexed. It was the doctor's first encounter with Tony's condition, which was called an imperforate anus. In other words, Tony's intestinal organs were intact, but they stopped short; there was no rectal opening. Surgery to create an opening was absolutely necessary and needed to be done right away, the doctor explained, or the baby would die.

Tony was born at 2:58 in the afternoon. By 4:30 that same day, he was in the operating room where the surgeons performed delicate colostomy surgery on the newborn. It would be the first of nearly a dozen operations the boy would face before he would enter kindergarten. One of those operations occurred when Tony was about nine months old. Doctors tried to create a more normal anal opening, only to discover that he had only 10 percent sphincter muscle control.

Uncertain about what to do next, doctors refashioned a second colostomy. A couple of years later, his colostomy was reversed once more in an attempt to allow Tony to eliminate normally. Even though he had matured some, he still lacked enough muscle control and, again, he was forced to go back to having a colostomy.

For several years, there were attempts at reconstructive surgery, all the while trying to determine if Tony would ever develop the sphincter control he needed. In the meantime, none of the ostomy pouching systems available at the time worked for little Tony, and he was forced to wear diapers into his preschool years. (That has since changed, and today ConvaTec manufactures "Little Ones" especially designed for young kids.) As he got older, he switched to Pull-ups.

What does a little boy do who has no bowel control? How could he comprehend, being so young and unaware, that his physical condition often disturbed people?

But somehow he knew, so Tony did what any child would do in a similar situation: instead of playing with friends outside, he stayed indoors and played alone. He avoided most physical activity and never spent the night with friends. As he got older, Tony began to understand he was different.

One day, when the children in his kindergarten class wanted to know why Tony had "special bathroom privileges," Tony's kindergarten teacher asked him if he wanted to talk about it to the class. Tony said no at first but a few days later, he changed his mind. That day, during "Show and Tell," he stood up and began to talk.

"I have an im-per-for-ate anus," the five-year-old boy explained, enunciating each syllable for the solemn-faced children sitting in a circle around him. "That means I don't have any muscle to hold my poop in. That's why I have to wear this." He presented a Pull-up for his little classmates to see. Tony's teacher, who happened to be a friend of his mother, was touched by how brave Tony was being. Later she told Cindy, "He took the mystery out of it and made it easier for all of us to understand why he needed to do certain things that other kids didn't need to do."

But Tony's third-grade teacher didn't have the same empathy. Instead, she ridiculed the boy for his incontinence, one time pulling him out in the hallway and shaking him after he had had another "accident." Tony's parents still seethe over the incident. "Normally I support teachers," said Tony's mother, an elementary schoolteacher herself, "but this was wrong. The next day I was back at school raising a ruckus, standing up for Tony's rights to the teacher and the principal."

Tony's father agreed that the teacher's behavior was totally uncalled for and embarrassing to his son. "It fed the fire, as far as peer pressure was concerned," he explained.

Partly due to this incident, the Bells realized things had to change for Tony. They discussed their options with Tony's pediatrician and decided that their son needed a permanent colostomy if he was to have any chance of a normal childhood. For his parents, who had been hoping to postpone the decision so Tony could make it on his own when he was older, the realization was agonizing. It meant not only having to tell their son that he would need yet another surgery, but also explaining to him that he would have to live with a colostomy for the rest of his life. They wondered if they were doing the right thing.

Tony's first response, when informed of his parents' decision, was to dig his heels in and refuse. The thought of another surgery was frightening to him. "I was having nightmares about hospitals," he recalls. "I can still smell the gas they used to put me to sleep. I didn't want to go back. But then they explained, 'Tony, you have a decision. You can either go through life wearing diapers and having one embarrassing situation after another, or you can have this colostomy.' When they assured me that my life would be significantly improved with the colostomy, I finally agreed."

Nine-year-old Tony walked into the hospital for the last time three weeks later. He walked in carrying a large, stuffed teddy bear hoping—believing—life would be much better when it was all over. And it was. But it would take a while for him to figure that out.

Trying to Get the Hang of It

He hated the ostomy appliance at first. The nurses

tried to teach him how to care for it, but he didn't want to hear it. In the beginning, his mother did most of the work changing the faceplate and making sure the skin around the stoma was properly cared for. For her it was a way she could finally help her precious little boy and she didn't mind at all.

As Tony got stronger and healed from the surgery his strong-willed nature took over and he began to get the hang of it. Pretty soon, he was doing the changing while his mother stood back and supervised. By the time school started, Tony was like the new kid on the block.

"Talk about a life-changing experience," says Tony, who is attending college these days at Fort Hays State University in Hays, Kansas. "I went from not going out of the house and having to carry two changes of clothes wherever I went, to buzzing around on my bike, walking two miles to the fishing pond, even helping my dad out on the farm. I was totally free to do what I wanted for the first time in my life!"

Summer ended and school started. Now in the fourth grade, Tony arrived that first day wearing shorts and tennis shoes, clothes he'd never been able to wear before. Until then, he'd always been worried about accidents and needed to wear dark jeans or sweat pants.

"Things went well until the end of the day," he remembers smiling ruefully. "It was the last hour of school, and my bag must have been pretty full. Since the colostomy was still fairly new to me, I hadn't quite gotten the hang of when to empty it. I was up on the monkey bars and somehow slipped and fell and landed flat on my stomach. Unfortunately, the pressure on the bag must have caused the clip to pop off. All of a sudden I could feel the warm contents of the bag running down my leg and into my shoe. I remember crying and frantically looking for the recess teacher. By then all the kids saw what had happened and began laughing at me. I was so embarrassed I wanted to die."

Tony went home in tears and angrily confronted his parents. "I thought you said life would be better after surgery," he blurted out between sobs. Heartbroken, his parents tried to comfort him and explain that it would take time, that life sometimes has a strange way of teaching us things. Besides, how much worse could it get?

But things did get worse. From that fourth grade until his sophomore year in high school, Tony was known as "the kid with the disability" or "Mr. Rubber Maid." He survived by hanging out with one friend, a kid named Dustin. "He was the school nerd, and I was the school retard," says Tony, doing his best to laugh about it now, but obviously still pained by memories of cruel taunting and bullying.

Tony's freshman year in high school was the worst. He had a gym teacher that seemed to enjoy making fun of him. Tony did his best to "grin and bear it," but things came to a head one day when he had an accident in class and the teacher took the opportunity to belittle Tony in front of his classmates. "He said I'd never grow up to be anything, since I obviously couldn't even use the toilet like normal people." Making matters worse, the gym teacher's son, who was Tony's age, began to pick on Tony as well.

Tony took it and took it, trying to do the right thing, but he never told his parents about what was going on in school. At night, he'd often cry himself to sleep wondering if his nightmare would ever end. Through it all he struggled to focus on what his father had tried to teach him; that except for this one problem, he was normal, and there was nothing he couldn't do if he really set his mind to it. His dad kept reminding him that if he let this one thing get him down, then being down was his own choice.

Tony wanted to make a different choice, and finally one day he did. It came during an art class, which he shared with his gym teacher's son. During a moment when the instructor had stepped out of the room, the boy started in on Tony. This time Tony didn't back down. With years of pent up anger, he stood up and looked his accuser straight in the eye.

"I can't help the way I was born," he sneered at the boy. The room fell silent. "Just like you can't help it that you were born with crooked teeth. I don't make fun of you. What gives you the right to make fun of me?"

Unfazed, the boy replied, "Hey, if I want to, I can take my pencil and poke you right in your shit bag."

Tony met his gaze, unflinching. "Go ahead," he challenged.

The boy leaped at Tony, and in the ensuing melee, he stabbed his pencil at Tony's abdomen. Then he struck pay dirt. The contents of the bag oozed out all over Tony's shirt and pants as the boy hooted and hollered with delight. Tony used every ounce of self-control to keep from taking his anger and beating his tormentor to a pulp. Instead, he picked up his things, left the room, and headed straight for the principal's office.

Between clenched teeth, he explained what had just happened—including the problem with his gym teacher.

The principal went into action, suspending the boy and firing the teacher, but it was too little and much too late. Embarrassed and hurt, Tony refused to return to a school where everything and everybody would remind him of one of the worst days of his life. Instead, he transferred to the high school where his dad taught, thirty miles away. It was there that things began to change.

From the beginning, he knew things were going to be different at the new school because the students didn't know Tony's health history. He felt good that he had finally stood up for himself and made a clean break. Through that experience, Tony grew up and became a little closer to learning what he was really made of.

He started wearing his Stetson hat his sophomore year. Rather than ridiculing him, the students at Santa Fe Trail High School admired Tony, calling him "Cowboy." By then he had been rodeoing for four years and had already become addicted to the adrenaline rush that comes when "it's just man against beast." He was only fifteen years old now, but Tony was wiser beyond his years. "People in rodeo didn't care what your limitations were," he explains. "They knew that if you're out there trying, you deserve all the respect in the world."

For a young man who had spent most of his adolescent life humiliated by the taunts and barbs of people who never thought he'd amount to anything, he was proving a lot of folks wrong.

Giving the Signal

Tony could've been thinking all this as he climbed into the chute and eased himself down onto the two tons of raw furry he was about to battle. Instead, his mind was clear as his heart pounded, and the adrenaline started to flow. He fixed his eyes on the space between the animal's horns, wrapped his legs around the huge chest of the bull and, with his right hand, clenched the rope. With his left hand slightly raised, he paused for a moment and then nodded to the cowboy holding the gate. In an instant the chute gate was flung open, and the bull charged into the arena.

Tony held on with all his might and, for eight glorious seconds, had the thrill of his life. Tony has been riding life like that ever since, and he doesn't plan to stop anytime soon.

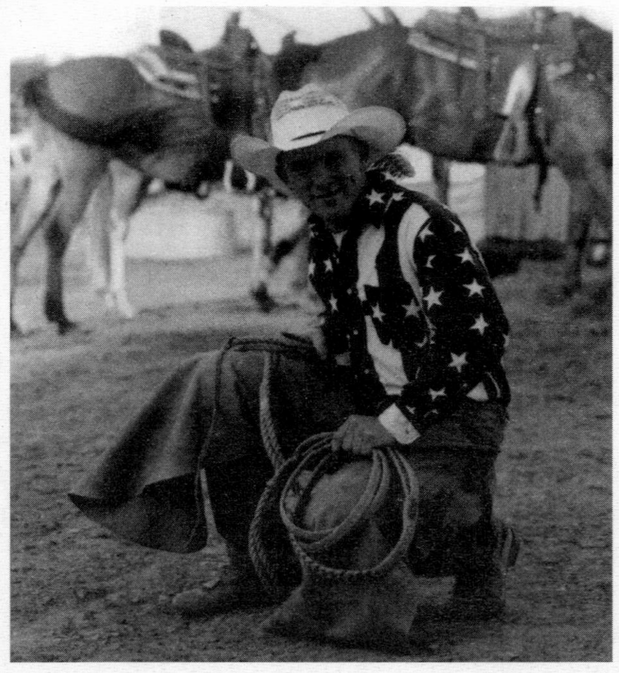

Despite being born with an imperforate anus, Tony Bell's tenacity and courage earned him a bull-riding scholarship to Fort Hays State University in Kansas and the respect of anyone who meets him.

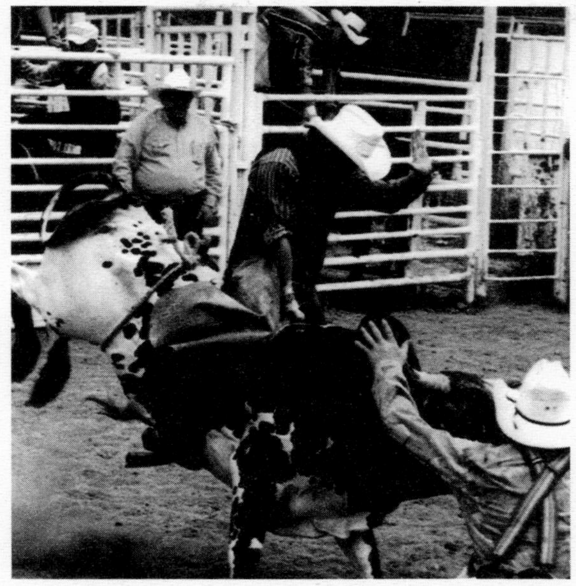

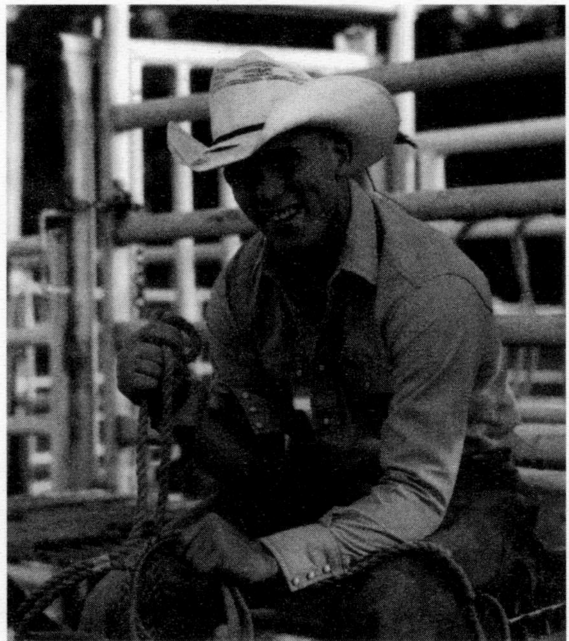

Ride'em, Cowboy! Bull rider Tony Bell has demonstrated his toughness in rodeos throughout the Midwest, taking on two-ton beasts and hanging on for dear life.

Because he was born without an opening in his rectum, Tony required multiple surgeries and was forced to wear diapers for almost ten years. It was the cruel comments from unsympathetic classmates and teachers that sometimes made riding a bull seem easier than going to school.

SCORCHED DREAM?

MICHAEL NASH

AGE

40

HOMETOWN

San Diego, California

MEDICAL SITUATION

In the midst of a demanding career as a firefighter, Michael's chronic ulcerative colitis forced him to undergo ostomy surgery.

Summer, 1996. Atlanta, Georgia. It was the Olympics, where athletes from all over the world competed for glory and medals and the pride of their nations. It was where stories of great triumph and anguishing despair would unfold. Where months and years of training would come down to a few hundredths of a second and leave the competitors exhilarated or crushed. On the largest stage in the world the excitement was intense and the pressure almost palpable.

Summer, 1996. The year a bomb exploded in Olympic Centennial Park, leaving two people dead and over 100 injured. Was it the work of international terrorists or a lone madman? A fascinated world watched, absorbed by the unfolding drama, wondering how it would all end. There was nothing like the Olympic theater to attract the eyes and ears of an eager world, citizens of each country watching with national pride on the line. During those few short weeks, everyday life seems to come to a standstill, and everything takes a backseat to the intensity and the grandeur of the Olympics.

Summer, 1996. Beneath the surface of the pageantry and the spectacle taking place that hot, muggy summer, another drama reaches its apex—the story of one man's personal dream nearly shattered by chronic disease. It's the story not of an Olympic athlete or a deranged bomber, but of a young firefighter from San Diego, California.

While the athletes rested comfortably in the Olympic village, Michael Nash hunkered down in a tent not far away, awaiting orders. He was on edge, ready and anxious to respond when the call came. Part of an elite Urban Search and Rescue Team, Michael was one of fifty-six men whose bodies were as fit and whose minds as sharp as any Olympic competitor. They were the best in the business, selected from units all across the nation.

While being in Atlanta as part of the USAR Team was quite an accomplishment, for Michael it was way more than that. It represented the pinnacle of a dream that he figured had gone up in flames four months earlier when, lying in a hospital bed in the aftermath of intestinal surgery, he awoke to news he believed would end his hard-won career as a firefighter.

The Seed of a New Dream

Many kids dream about becoming a fireman when they grow up. Not Michael. He always wanted to be a football player—a quarterback. When, that dream didn't materialize, he ended up settling for construction. Steady work, but not what you'd call exhilarating. One day, out on a job site banging nails, a friend talked about how neat it would be to be in the fire service. That one discussion planted the seed of a new dream, one that would take over five years of intense study and night classes and getting into top physical shape while still working his day job to germinate.

"Few people understand how grueling and competitive it is to become a firefighter," Michael explains. "For every opening, there are several hundred people knocking on the door for that position. It's ruthless!" Nevertheless, after years of determined study and personal tenacity, the door finally opened. Michael was in.

"I remember the day I learned I had been hired as a firefighter," he says. "It was shortly before my twenty-ninth birthday and my dad threw me a party. I was ecstatic." Michael celebrated with the rest of his family and friends, but one nagging thought dampened the evening. He'd been having stomach problems for five years—cramping, diarrhea—nothing he couldn't handle, but still, a nuisance, a discomfort, and a concern. Doctors thought at first the problem was an ulcer and treated him accordingly. The symptoms lessened, even disappeared. But then they returned. There was more pain. More testing before the diagnosis came in: ulcerative colitis. Michael was twenty-six years old at the time.

That night at the party, Michael's emotions fluctuated like the flickering candles on his birthday cake. Before him, like an immense sea, surging with possibilities and new challenge, loomed this incredible opportunity, this dream come true. Anchored to him, however, dragging him down, was the reality that his body was not healthy. Michael was about to enter a profession that would not only take an incredible amount of physical stamina, but would also require immediate response when an alarm went off. Yet from one moment to the next, he had no idea what to expect from his impaired intestines. Would he be stricken with a bout of diarrhea in the middle of a midnight call? Would his physical limitations hinder his abilities, hamper his effectiveness, put at risk the men he was called to serve with? Was it right for him to enter a profession in which duty depended on reflex, stamina, and strength?

These questions and more swirled in his head that night, but he wasn't about to be deterred. He'd come too far, worked too hard. Somehow he'd manage. Who knew? Maybe the disease would become a non-issue. He had learned that ulcerative colitis can be chronic and sometimes require surgery; or, it can present only as flare-ups that can be managed medically. Maybe he'd be one of the lucky ones. With a mixture of anticipation and apprehension, Michael embarked upon his first year as a firefighter.

It was an intense year, a probationary time, during which he could be terminated for anything from incompetence to inappropriate behavior to poor health. Perhaps it was a latent period of the disease, or maybe it was sheer determination and mind over matter. Whatever it was, Michael got through that first year without seeing a doctor and officially became a firefighter.

Michael didn't stop there. Two years after embarking on his new career, Michael Nash was selected to become a member of the San Diego Urban Search and Rescue Team. The team is made up of building engineers, paramedics, doctors, rescue dogs and their trainers, rescue technicians, and rescue specialists, and is usually deployed during major disasters like earthquakes, bombings, floods, or tornadoes. Currently there are only twenty-eight elite search and rescue teams in the United States, eight of which are in California. Michael Nash, ulcerative colitis and all, served on one.

Those first few years on the job were everything he had hoped they would be, and more. A typical day at the station might result in ten or more calls, mostly in response to medical emergencies or traffic accidents, but occasionally to battle a structural blaze or wildfire. The job was both physically challenging and mentally satisfying. Nevertheless, those early years weren't easy.

Michael's health problems had returned. He didn't talk about them with his co-workers, and he never complained. Somehow he managed to get by without allowing his illness to interfere with his work, though there were some close calls. Once, while fighting a brush fire, he almost lost control of his bowels and had to literally squat in the bushes to relieve himself. Still, he persevered . . . after all this was his dream, what he had lived for, and he wasn't about to give in to a "stomach ache."

But one day there came a breaking point when no amount of willpower or denial could change what was happening to his body. Nearly five years into his career, he found himself in the hospital following an especially severe flare-up. Suddenly it became clear that he could no longer will it away. He couldn't take a pill to cure it, and he could no longer mask the symptoms or hide from the impact the colitis was having on his life. It became apparent, even to Michael, that the disease wasn't going to quietly fade away.

Not long after this bout, Michael's physician suggested he see a surgeon. His heart sank. Surgery—the removal of his bowel? Surely, Michael thought, that would mean the end of his fire-fighting career. It was a huge decision, but one that he knew he had to come to grips with.

So he attacked the problem much like he would a fire. He didn't just rush in blindly, preferring to survey the situation carefully before acting. He contacted the United Ostomy Association, read as much as he could about what it would be like to live with an ostomy, and he even spoke to several people who had had the surgery.

In his search, he stumbled on something unexpected and hopeful—a fellow firefighter who had had ostomy surgery and returned to the job! Could it be? Was there really still a chance . . . a light at the end of the tunnel? Suddenly the possibility of surgery became less daunting. And when Michael's surgeon informed him he probably wouldn't need a permanent ostomy but a J-Pouch instead, that sealed it. Michael decided to go ahead with the surgery.

Galvanized by the possibility of putting all the years of illness and discomfort behind him once and for all, Michael sprang into action. He scheduled the surgery and arranged for an eight-to-ten week recovery period at work. Everyone was excited. Michael's wife, Michelle, completely supported the decision and looked forward to finally getting her husband back. His co-workers and even his Fire Chief wished him well. Everything was set. Only one more hurdle, he thought, succumbing to the anesthesia. One more. . . .

A Detour

The first thing he remembers as he emerged from his drugged stupor was Michelle sitting beside him, holding his hand. Everything was foggy, blurred. He couldn't focus his eyes. But he knew Michelle's touch, her familiar smell, and the sound of her voice. As he slowly struggled to regain consciousness he began to sense that something wasn't quite right.

"They couldn't do it," she said softly. "The J-Pouch. They tried, but they couldn't do it. . . . "

The surgeon entered the room just then. Michael tried to speak, but he couldn't form the words. The doctor spoke, instead. He was matter-of-fact. "You're going to have the permanent ileostomy, Michael. I'm sorry. But don't worry. You'll be just fine. We'll help you get used to it, show you how to take care of yourself. In no time at all, you'll be leading a normal, healthy life." He patted Michael's shoulder, said goodbye for now, then left. He had other patients to take care of.

Like a match casually tossed on dry kindling, Michael saw his dream to return to the force suddenly ignite and get consumed in a blazing inferno. He lay on the bed, Michelle still holding his hand, not knowing what to think or say. Slowly what the surgeon had just said sank in and he began to sob . . . deep gut-wrenching sobs that he couldn't stifle even though they caused his new long abdominal incision to hurt horribly. It was nothing like the pain that was breaking his heart.

Michael spent his next days in the Intensive Care Unit, fighting a post-operative infection. Besides the normal nursing care he received, he also had stoma nurses showing him how to change the appliance. It was their goal not only to take care of him but also to get him to learn to do it by himself. At one point he tried but after a few seconds, gave up. "I can't do this," he shouted angrily at the nurse. "I hate this thing. I'll never be able to do it by myself." Then he broke down.

Later that day, Michael was moved from the ICU to a regular room on the surgical recovery floor. He was in pain physically and at the end of his rope emotionally. So when an intern accidentally spilled his urinal all over him, he wondered if he had made the right choice to have surgery. He wondered if he was going to have to endure a lifetime of indignities.

Michael shared his new room with another patient who had also just undergone abdominal surgery. Lon had an upbeat attitude and joked often with the nurses. Although Michael was in no mood to talk, slowly Lon's cheerful outlook began to affect Michael. Though his spirits didn't lift immediately, as the pain subsided and he slowly began to heal, his strength began to return, and with it, his competitive nature. By the time he was released from the hospital, he had made a very important decision. This surgery was not going to ruin his life.

He had come through a very difficult ordeal and survived. Suddenly, he had a whole new appreciation for life and was determined to make the most of it. He learned to take one day at a time and, for the moment, he was just happy to be alive!

With his new attitude, it wasn't long before Michael began to get the hang of changing his ostomy appliance and the way his body reacted to food. He could anticipate when his bag would fill up and knew he needed to empty it before he went out for any extended period. It was awkward at first, and he had his share of frustrating moments, but with time and practice he slowly began to settle into a routine.

In the back of his mind, however, was the uncertainty of his future. It was one thing to learn to change his bag in the comfort and privacy of his own home—but what about the fire station? What would the guys think? Could he ever really do his job the way he needed to? He had opted for the surgery because he was told he would end up with a J-pouch and not a permanent ileostomy. Now all bets were off, and Michael wondered if his firefighting days were over.

Desperate for help he called a good friend and fellow firefighter, Rick, who knew all that he had been through.

"What am I going to do about work?" Michael asked almost desperately.

"What do you mean 'What am I going to do about my work'?" Rick retorted. "What's the big deal? You've got a job to do. We miss you, and we need you back."

Michael protested, but Rick was adamant. "Name one reason why you can't come back."

"Other than the fact that my belly was just sliced open and I have a crap bag attached to my gut?" Michael responded angrily.

"Besides that," Rick answered.

Rick made it seem so simple, but Michael wasn't sure. It wasn't until Steve Miller, the president of the local firefighters union, entered the picture that Michael finally came around. Steve was an ex-Marine who had not earned the nickname "Bulldog" for nothing. He took Michael's case personally and began banging on the doors of Human Resources and talking to the Fire Chief in person, insisting, in no uncertain terms, that Nash was coming back to work.

Steve Miller had everyone convinced but Michael Nash himself. When Steve heard that Michael was still having doubts, the Bulldog turned on Michael.

"Nash, you'd better not let me down," he snarled. "I've gone to bat for you."

That was just the kick in the rear that Michael needed. He realized it was now up to him. The way had been paved, and he didn't want to disappoint all the people who believed in him. Besides, he loved being a firefighter.

His first task was to get back into shape. But where do you start when simply getting out of bed was an agonizing challenge? His abdominal muscles had been sliced completely through, and the doctors reminded him not to do anything strenuous for a while. The muscles needed time to knit back together.

But Michael could walk. So he made one painful shuffling step after another. Day after day and week after week he walked. He was determined to get better.

Each day he walked a little farther, did a little more and, gradually, his strength returned. By the time eight weeks had passed, Michael was fit enough—and excited—about returning to work.

When he did return, it was as if he'd never left. Although he wasn't 100 percent yet, he was out there, working. The guys saw that he could keep up and accepted him. The dream was still alive.

Michael had been back only a short time when his battalion chief approached him about the possibility of working at the upcoming Olympics. Michael had been on the Urban Search and Rescue Team for nearly five years and, because of the constant threat of terrorists, the teams would be needed in Atlanta.

Prior to his surgery, Michael had known about the possibility of going to the Olympics and had often thought how special it would be protecting athletes from all over the world . . . but that was then. Since his operation, he had tried to keep from thinking about Atlanta, preferring to focus on doing everything he could to get back to being a regular firefighter.

"Michael, you're the most qualified guy we have for this job. Can you do it?" His battalion chief continued.

Could it be? Was there really a chance he could go? His heart began pounding.

Accepting the opportunity would be a tremendous privilege but also a huge personal challenge. Was he ready? The team would be roughing it, camping out, and using outdoor bathroom facilities. There'd be no privacy. He was still getting used to his ileostomy pouch. What would happen if there were leaks and accidents?

Then there was the team. A few guys from his area knew about the surgery, but what about the new guys he would meet? Would they be as understanding? He wasn't sure. He had his doubts.

Then, something occurred to him. His fire chief knew all that Michael had just gone through. He knew about the ostomy and, yet, he was still asking him to go. He wasn't looking at Michael's limitations; he was looking at Michael's qualifications.

Buoyed by his battalion chief's confidence in him, Michael agreed to go. It turned into one of the highlights of his career, almost convincing him that maybe—just maybe—he really could come all the way back and become a firefighter again.

Not long after he returned from Atlanta, Michael

found himself battling not one but three structural fires in a single day. Only firefighters realize how unlikely such a scenario is. Yet there he was—four months after waking up on a hospital bed to life-changing surgery and what he thought was the scorching of his dream—at the helm of a screaming fire truck, nerves taut, muscles strained, racing from one fire to the next. It was the most physically grueling day of his entire career.

Driving home that night with the Chief, Michael couldn't help but marvel. Turning to his boss, he said matter-of-factly, "Hey, Chief. Look what happened today. I just went to three working structure fires and kept up with all the guys!" He leaned back in his seat, closed his eyes and grinned.

The chief glanced at Michael for a moment before looking back to the road. "Welcome back," he said proudly. "We all knew you could do it . . . and now you know it, too."

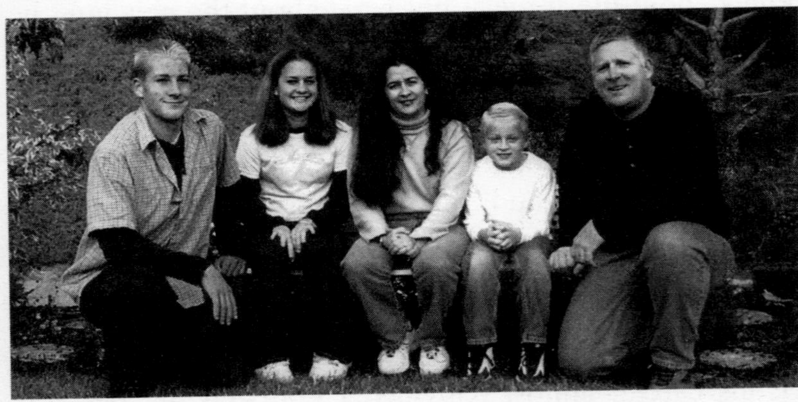

With his wife, Michelle, and their three children in his corner, Michael Nash survived a difficult battle with ulcerative colitis and resumed his firefighting career. Remarkably, just a few short months after his operation, he realized a dream and was picked as a member of the Urban Search and Rescue Team for the 1996 Olympic Games in Atlanta.

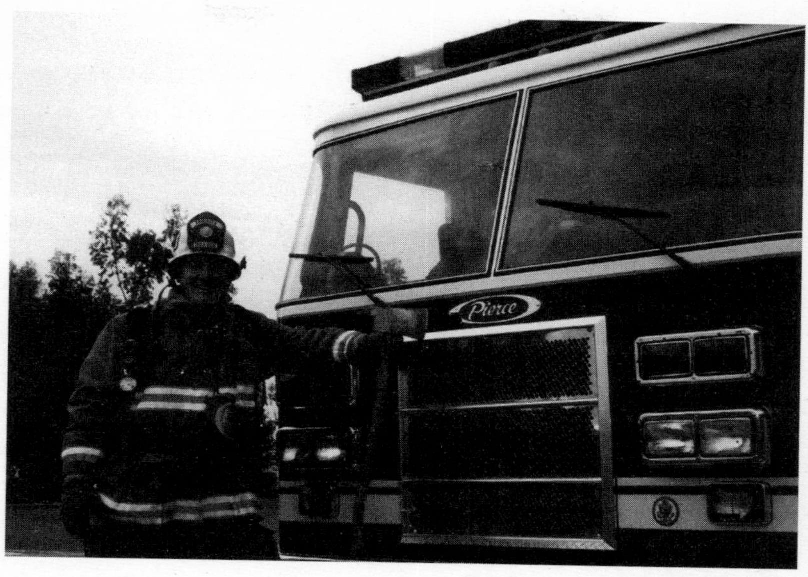

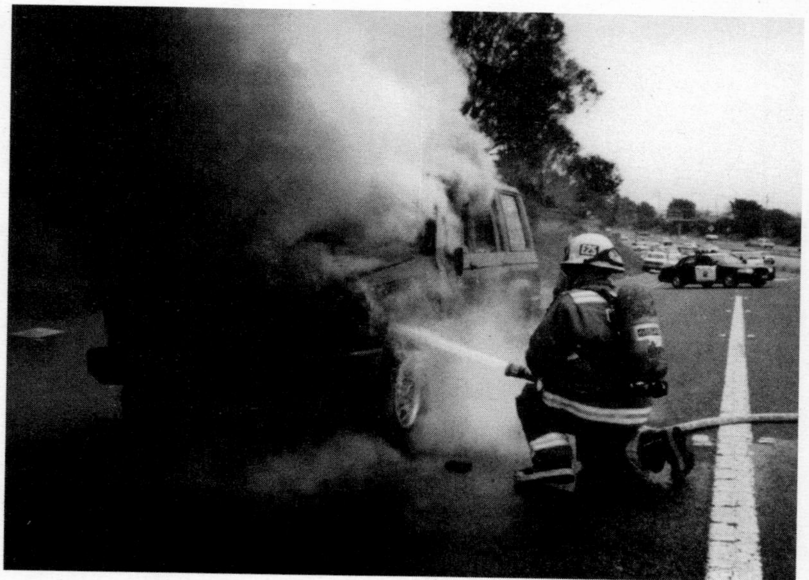

When you're a firefighter, you never know when the emergency call will come. For Michael Nash, it doesn't matter—he'll be ready.

Still Smelling Those Roses

OTTO GRAHAM

AGE

80

HOMETOWN

Sarasota, Florida

MEDICAL SITUATION

At the age of fifty-six, following a stellar career as an NFL quarterback, Otto was diagnosed with colon cancer and needed colostomy surgery.

In the huddle, the quarterback meets the gaze of his teammates, and then he calls the play. There's a fleeting sense of camaraderie and respect before the huddle breaks and the players hustle into position. Then the ball is snapped.

The quarterback takes his customary seven-step drop, eyes the field, sensing if not seeing the frenzied conflict taking place in his periphery. He knows that he has only a few seconds before big defensive linemen will break through his protection and try to knock him senseless.

Quick wits, sharp reflexes, and a receiver streaking down the field converge in a split-second decision when the quarterback launches the ball into sky. As the deep throw spirals through the air, fans rise to their feet. The receiver lays out in a full stretch for the perfect throw and makes a finger-tip catch, getting his feet down in bounds in the back corner of the end zone. Touchdown!

For Otto Graham, who flung hundreds of passes back in the late 1940s and 1950s, this was a common occurrence. During his heyday, he emerged as one of the finest quarterbacks in the history of professional football, and those old enough to remember haven't forgotten "Automatic Otto."

Otto played in the days when football players wore helmets with no face guards, and it was a badge of honor to have a couple of your front teeth knocked out. Though Otto never did lose a tooth, it was a twelve-inch gash from his lip up his cheek (from a nasty blow during a game with the San Francisco 49ers, resulting in twenty-six stitches) that brought about a revolutionary change in football headgear. His coach, Paul Brown of the Cleveland Browns, improvised a two-inch wide Plexiglas face guard for Otto after that injury, making Otto the first player to ever wear a facemask. It wasn't long before facemasks became required headgear—that's how far back Otto Graham goes.

A Career Begins

There aren't enough superlatives to describe this legendary Hall of Famer. The "greatest of all players," as Coach Brown has described him, consistently still ranks as one of the top passers of all time. He earned the nickname "Automatic Otto" way back in his sophomore year at college when, as a scholarship basketball player at Northwestern University in Evanston, Illinois, not far from his hometown in Waukegan, Otto Everett Graham, Jr., the second son of two schoolteachers, was recruited to play basketball at Northwestern, with football and baseball as side lines. Otto's nickname came ostensibly as a result of his precision shooting on the basketball court and passing on the gridiron, but also because, as Otto's eldest son, Duey, puts it, "Everything was accurate and automatic to Dad. He came through every time, whether he was making a lay-up or throwing a touchdown pass."

Otto was one of the first—and the last—three-sport stars at Northwestern, where he was also a standout on the baseball diamond. It was a grueling schedule, wearing leather cleats one day and canvas sneakers the next. Nevertheless, he excelled. As a college junior on the football team, Otto set a Big Ten record, completing 89 of 182 passes for 1,092 yards. The following year, Otto was All-American in both football and basketball, and he was good enough in the latter sport to play one year of pro basketball for the Rochester Royals before turning to professional football.

Though athletics was obviously a huge part of Otto Graham's college career, he maintained the family tradition by majoring in education and minoring in music, playing the French horn and coronet in a brass sextet and the violin in his college orchestra. He didn't, however, follow in his parents' footsteps and become a music teacher as he had originally intended. In spite of his phenomenal athletic career, he will tell anyone who asks and even those who don't that giving up music after college is his biggest regret. He would trade all the trophies he ever earned as an athlete, he says, to have stuck with his music.

After college, Otto did a two-year pre-flight stint in the Navy, and it was around this time that he married his college sweetheart, Beverly Jean Collinge. Otto recalls practicing his "passes" one evening by tossing peas at the table where Beverly sat with a friend. He was aiming for Beverly's blouse. Compared to most of the girls, Otto says, Beverly was the "most wonderful." They married shortly after he was discharged from the Navy.

Otto's history with the Cleveland Browns began with a bit of controversy. The American Football League was not yet formed, and the Detroit Lions of the NFL had just drafted Otto. Unbeknownst to Otto, Ohio State coach Paul Brown, impressed by Otto's college football career, was forming what would become the Cleveland Browns in a new pro football league called the All-American Football Conference. The athlete that Coach Brown had pegged for his quarterback was none other than Otto Graham.

Coach Brown contacted Otto, told him about the new league, and offered him an unprecedented amount of money at the time: $7,500 for the first year, with a $1,000 signing bonus. Otto couldn't believe his good fortune, so he accepted the offer—the best decision he ever made. "I would have been a different football player if I'd gone to Detroit," he says now. "You'd never have heard of me. I was lucky to sign with Coach Brown. He gets 90 percent of the credit for who I am."

The Brown-Graham relationship proved to be practically indestructible. The Cleveland Browns dominated professional football in the late '40s, winning all four AAFC championship games before merging with the NFL. And even then, when pundits assumed the greater NFL would overwhelm the weaker start-up league, the Browns stunned everyone by beating the Los Angeles Rams in the NFL championship game during their inaugural season in 1950.

And that was only the beginning. All told, during his ten-year pro football career, Otto led the Cleveland Browns to seven championships before retiring in 1955. He was selected the Most Valuable Player five times during his tenure with the Browns; was recently named one of the top 100 Athletes of the Millennium by ESPN; was among the top six football players of all time identified by *Sports Illustrated*; and was named the sixth-ranked gridiron star of all time by *Sport Magazine*.

Remarkably self-effacing for a legend, Otto dismisses the accolades. "My one claim to fame," insists the eighty-year-old retiree, who spends his twilight years driving balls on a golf course in Sarasota, Florida, where he lives with Beverly, "is that Vince Lombardi replaced me as coach and general manager of the Washington Redskins in 1969."

He chuckles as he recalls the day he heard the news. "I was out in California playing golf, and I read in the paper that Lombardi was coming in to replace me. I was fired!" Graciously conceding that it was probably a good decision, Otto adds, "I was a good coach, but I did have one fault. I was too nice a guy. Even my assistant coaches told me I was too nice."

Otto shakes his head. "Listen," he says, as if needing to remind himself of those days when he was coaching. "You don't say 'please' and 'thank you' to these guys. You've got to chew them out. There's no question—I could have been a better coach if I'd been tougher."

Onrushing Health Problems

"Soft" isn't the first word that comes to mind when you talk with Otto Graham. In fact, mention Vince Lombardi to him after all these years, and he's spitting nails again. "Lombardi was a great coach, no doubt about it, but he was *stupid* when it came to his health," says the six-foot octogenarian. Obviously not one to mince words, he adds, "I guess Lombardi thought he was invincible. I may not be a doctor, but I do think he diminished his chances of survival because he waited too long before seeking treatment."

Otto is referring to the rectal cancer that eventually killed Lombardi in 1970. The subject is particularly poignant to Otto Graham, who himself was diagnosed with the same form of cancer in 1977. Yet here he is, twenty-five years later, and not only is Otto alive, but he is alive and well and clearly none the worse for his wear. "You know what I liked best about being in the hospital," he confides. "I liked it when the nurses took me to the bathroom. Now I always tell people not to try and goose me," he continues, "because there's nothing there!"

He laughs at his favorite joke, one he repeats at banquets and high school campuses, where he freely discusses the life-saving colostomy surgery in which his colon and rectum were removed and left him wearing a colostomy pouch. "I tell young people, you've got to be smart," he says. "You may have God-given abilities, but you've also got to use your head. I learned very quickly in sports that it doesn't matter what you look like. It's the lessons you learn in life that matter. So you can play ball—so what? What kind of a job do you do? What kind of a person are you?"

Back to Vince Lombardi. "He had symptoms, I'm sure," says Otto, obviously piqued. "But he kept putting off getting them checked, and then it was too late. There's no question that doctors could have saved his life." He pauses briefly, as if reminded of something from years ago. "Sure, surgery is frightening. But what's the alternative? If somebody would rather be dead than have surgery, then I have no sympathy for him or her."

Tough words, borne out of experience. Otto was fifty-six and coaching at the Coast Guard Academy in New London, Connecticut, when he discovered that he had colon cancer. But Otto didn't back away from the challenge. As the late *Los Angeles Times* sportswriter Jim Murray put it, ". . . he picked apart a zone defense few people can penetrate—cancer. It's a pass rush that won't let you stay in the pocket, the ultimate blitz." Otto's cancer might never have been detected but for the fact that the Coast Guard Academy required mandatory health check-ups. It was a combination of these check-ups and Otto being willing to discuss his symptoms that led to the diagnosis. Indeed, Otto credits early detection with the fact that he's even alive to talk about his cancer today. "Don't be a damn fool," he advises. "The odds are in your favor if you get it in time."

Otto was given only one option—surgery—and, true to form, he didn't blink. "I knew I had to get it done, so we did it quickly," he says. "There was nothing else to do. I didn't even think about what it would mean or what the future would hold."

In Otto's case, that future meant wearing a colostomy pouch. For some reason, though, Otto was unfazed by the prospect. "Dad's a realist," explains Duey Graham, who at age fifty-four is writing a biography of his father—something he believes should have been done a long time ago. "He's a black-and-white sort of a guy, not one to show his emotions." Speaking from his home in Boothbay, Maine, where he lives with his two cats and works as a sportswriter and novelist, Duey says that when Otto learned about the cancer and the need for ostomy surgery, he was matter-of-fact about it. "His response was, 'Okay, I've got cancer, and I'm going to have a colostomy. Let's get on with it.' "

It was, according to Beverly, vintage Otto Graham. "Otto's a team player," says his wife of over fifty years. "Whenever he lost a game, Otto felt like it was his fault, as if he had let his team down. As quarterback, he felt he had some control over the outcome. Cancer, on the other hand, wasn't something he could control. So when the time came for Otto to tell the family, it wasn't so difficult since he felt that he wasn't letting them down."

"A football player isn't great on his own," maintains Otto, elaborating on this idea of being a team player. "I don't care how good an athlete you are, a quarterback is nothing without his team. I need guys with good hands, blockers to give me the time to throw, and receivers to catch the ball. I could never have succeeded on my own. A quarterback is only as good as his coach and the players around him."

Close Family, Close Team

It's that team mentality, which Duey suspects was ingrained in Otto from years of musical training, that may explain why Otto was able to take the whole cancer experience in stride and ultimately kept him from being beaten down by this adversary. When the Graham family heard the news, like guards and tackles protecting their quarterback, they rallied to their parents' side. Otto and Beverly's youngest son David, who was earning his Master's degree at the time and living in Pennsylvania, left school and moved back to Washington D.C., where the surgery took place at Bethesda Naval Hospital. He would become Beverly's chauffeur, on call and available whenever she needed to be taken somewhere. Says Beverly, who stayed with a friend in the D.C. area during this period of time, "I was never alone. David was always there."

After Otto's release from the hospital, David's wife, Mary, quit her job, and the two of them moved in with his parents and offered to stay as long as they were needed. One of David's primary roles was to stave off the influx of visitors and well-wishers who continually dropped in. David and Mary ended up staying for almost a month before returning to Pennsylvania.

The "team" rallied again on a different level after Otto's normally unflagging optimism took a sack when, soon after his first surgery, Otto began to experience problems with the stoma. "They waited and waited for Dad to have a decent flow from the stoma," explains Duey, "but unfortunately, he had developed adhesions, which caused blockages."

Otto returned to the hospital and endured two more operations—the first to deal with the adhesions, the second to search for a missing sponge, which was later found folded in a sheet. Even after these surgeries, Otto still had problems with the stoma. "What had happened," says Beverly, "was that the stool had dried and turned into cement. Otto couldn't pass it, and he was getting sicker and sicker." The doctors gave Otto the equivalent of a very violent laxative—what Beverly describes as "blasting" the stoma. The entire family was present when the blockage finally cleared. Victory! The whole "team" celebrated right there in Otto's hospital room.

The dual surgeries, which came so quickly after the

initial colostomy, did to Otto's spirits what the first surgery couldn't do. "Until then, he'd always been positive and upbeat, but then Dad lost forty-five pounds throughout the entire ordeal," says Duey. "This time he was ready to give up. He was talking suicide. He wanted to die. This was so out of character for Dad because he's always been the ultimate winner."

Compounding Otto's discouragement was the fact that he was scheduled to play in Cy Laughter's Bogey Buster Golf Tournament, and he had been trying to get back into shape so he could play. The second hospitalization was a severe setback, and it sent Otto spiraling into a deep depression. His lowest moment came when, during a hospital visit from Beverly, he took all his anger and frustration out on his wife. "Basically, he just laid into her," says Duey. "Mom came home sobbing."

Knowing all that Beverly had endured up to this point, he and David got in the car, drove back to the hospital, and David chastised their father. It only took about a day—or until his next morphine shot, Duey says, laughing—before Otto was back to himself. As they drove home from the hospital later that week, Otto gazed at the passing scenery, then turned to Beverly and said, "I guess I need to smell the roses, because this sure looks good to me."

One month later, a weakened but recovered Otto was back in the saddle, playing the annual Bogey Buster's Golf Tournament with partners Gerald Ford, Don Shula, Ara Parsegian, and Cy Laughter. "That first hole they were playing a Scramble format," recalls Beverly, "and they used Otto's drive. His second shot was on the green, and he sank the putt for a birdie. Then he said, 'That's it—I'm through for the day.'"

Otto's team won the tournament.

Insisting that the cancer and ensuing surgery were merely "bumps in the road," Otto, who recently celebrated his fifty-sixth wedding anniversary with Beverly, says the operation that left him wearing an ostomy pouch didn't change his life too much. "I wouldn't go back to the old way of elimination for anything," he says, half-joking. "If you have to go to the bathroom, you need to excuse yourself and go to the bathroom. Me? I can just sit here."

The Two-Minute Warning

Just last year, Otto Graham was diagnosed with Alzheimer's disease. Yet even this last blitz isn't enough to vanquish the aging quarterback. Growing introspective, he says, "I've lived a full life. I have a wife in my corner. We've had a great life together. We raised three children and eight foster children. All told, there are sixteen grandchildren and two great-grandchildren.

"I could have given up. I could have said, Let's not do this surgery—I'd rather die. But that's not me. I don't give up. It's an uncertain future for all of us, but you've got to be smart. In sports, you've got to use your head, and you've got to use your head in life, too. I'm getting old. I'm eighty years old. I've got arthritis. My days of golf are limited. But hell, I've had a great life. And those roses still smell pretty good."

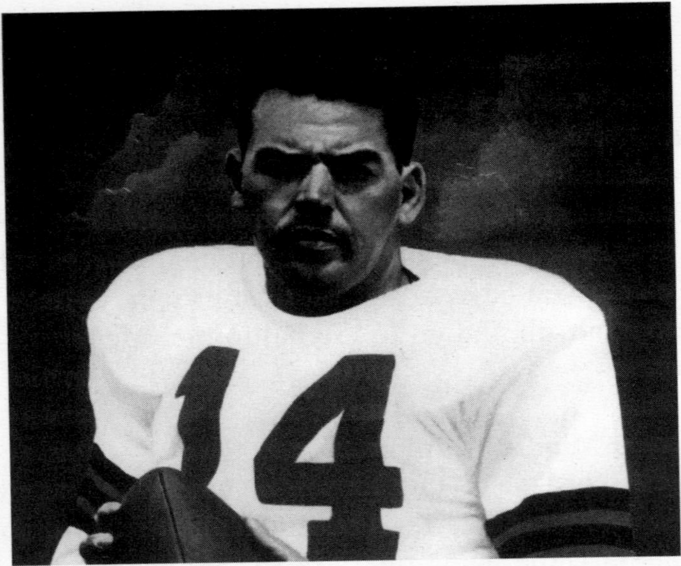

He played professional football in the early days before helmets had face guards, and you had to be tough. No one ever questioned Otto Graham's courage—or his ability—on the gridiron. This legendary NFL Hall of Fame quarterback was known as "Automatic Otto" during his playing days with the Cleveland Browns and established himself as one of the best quarterbacks ever to play the game.

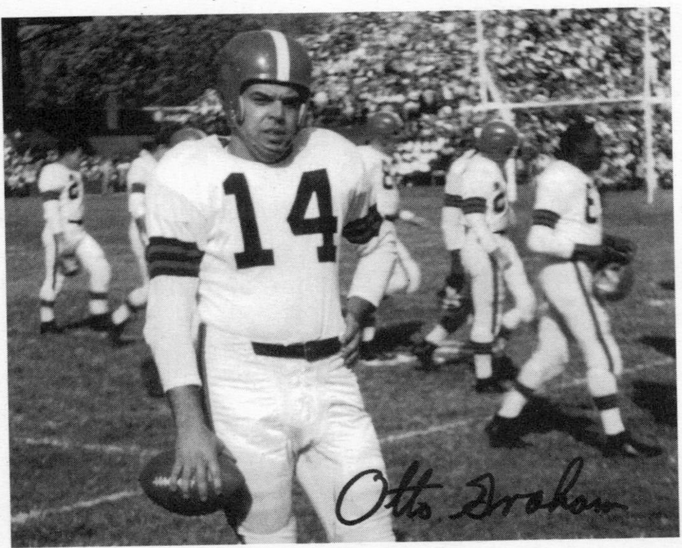

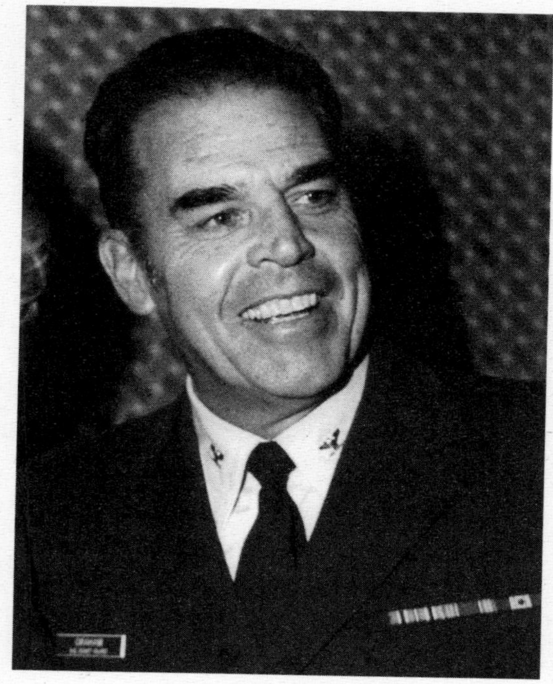

Nearly twenty years after he retired from the NFL, Otto was sacked one more time . . . this time by colon cancer. But with the same attitude that had seen him endure the toughest hits opposing linemen could deliver, Otto picked himself up after his colostomy surgery and returned to the active life he was enjoying before his operation.

Today, he's a hale and hardy eighty-year-old, still playing golf, and enjoying life with his wife, Beverly.

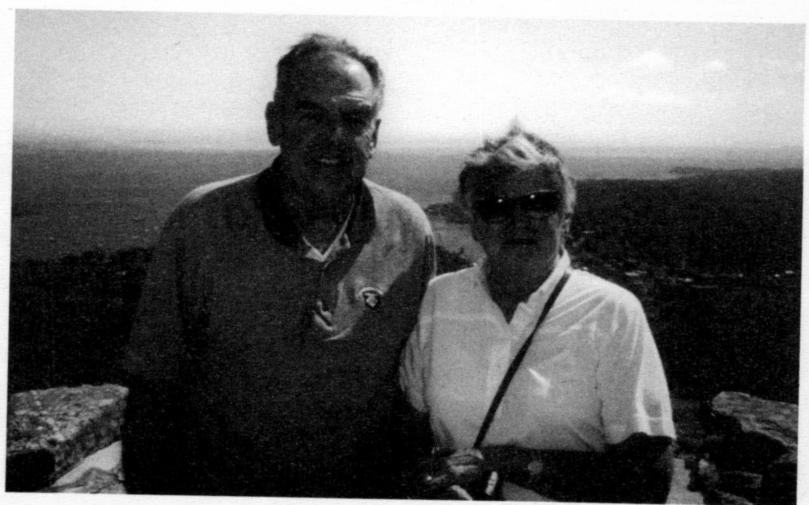

OSTO-MATES IN THE TRUE SENSE OF THE WORD

KEN & LINDA AUKETT

AGE
62 and 58

HOMETOWN
Westmont, New Jersey

MEDICAL SITUATION
He had an ileostomy in his early thirties, and she needed one in her late twenties . . . and then they met.

"You can't step twice in the same river."
— Heraclitus

Ken Aukett will tell you that he loves weather. Any kind of weather will do, but he especially loves extremes. Hurricanes. Earthquakes. Thunderstorms. Give Ken a nasty tempest, and he'll be satisfied.

In theory, that is. Ken had to rethink his passion for atmospheric fireworks on his honeymoon when he woke up somewhere in the Adirondacks and saw four inches of snow on the ground. It might not have been so bad, except that Ken wasn't your typical Eagle Scout. Roughing it loses a bit of its charm when your toes are cold.

That's not to say Ken wasn't prepared for weather. Call him "Eveready Ken" if you like, but in anticipation of his first canoe trip, he was all set. "One thing I learned as a kid," says the towering sixty-two-year old, "is *Be Prepared.*"

And prepared he was. Maybe too prepared. His

wife, Linda, thinks he went a little, shall we say, *overboard.* "Ken taught me the fine art of portage on that vacation," says Linda, wryly pointing out that everything they packed for their four-day honeymoon in the heart of the Adirondack Mountains—including air mattresses, rubber rain suits, and woolen pants—had to be hauled out of their canoe when setting up camp each night and lugged back to the canoe the following morning. Kitchen and food supplies were important as well—and we're not talking about eating beef jerky and pine nuts for dinner and breakfast. Ken included filet mignons, chicken breasts, and Bisquick pancake mix when he planned the gourmet menu.

All this camping paraphernalia was crammed inside their sixteen-foot canoe when they were on the move. Linda sat up front while Ken perched in the back, their gear piled so high that they could barely see each other. Linda, the bona fide camper of the two (she was a Girl Scout throughout her high school years), admits that she was somewhat mortified when the partially deflated air mattresses rounded off the pile, though she did appreciate the rain gear when the weather turned nasty.

Afternoon Breezes

Before we go much further, there's another story, one that Ken likes to tell over Linda's protestations. According to Ken, the first day of their October honeymoon was absolutely perfect. The autumn day was at its finest: invigoratingly crisp and cool, with bright sunlight glinting off the tranquil waters of Blue Mountain Lake like butterflies flitting in a field of bluebells and daylilies. The sapphire sky formed a magnificent palette against the woodland trees, now in their peak of splendor, and an afternoon breeze brushed softly through the array of leaves on display—Aspen, maple, tupelo, birch, hickory, cherry, oak, and elm.

Dazzling shades of wine-colored reds mingled gently with the softer, buttery hues of saffron, honey and gold. Like a banquet spread for royalty, the foliage surrounded them in a jubilee of color, and they feasted their eyes on tint and hue the way paupers would feast at a laden table. As the sun set and the moon rose over the little tent where the newlyweds spent their first evening as husband and wife, it was as though all of nature smiled upon them.

But, as New Englanders are fond of saying, "If you don't like the weather, wait a minute." With each passing day of their honeymoon, the weather conditions deteriorated, and meteorological hobbyist Ken got his fill of drama. The second night, torrential rains, heavy winds, thunder, lightning, and hail pummeled the couple as they huddled inside their tent and waited it out, both of them now grateful for the waterproof raingear and heavy-duty clothing that Ken had packed. On the third night temperatures dropped to 28 degrees, and here's the part of the story Ken likes to tell.

"Linda couldn't get warm," he says. "I let her use my down sleeping bag while I slept in the army bag, but she was still cold. We had brought some silver thermal blankets—the kind they use to wrap around runners at the end of a long race—and Linda decided to wrap up in one of those inside the down bag. Later that night, I woke up and heard all this commotion—a lot of noise and thumping. I reached for my flashlight, snapped it on, and there was Linda, stripping off all her clothes and jumping around inside the tent in her all-together. I thought, 'This must be some kind of ritual I don't know about.' But what had happened was, she had gotten so darned hot inside the down bag with the thermal blanket, she was drenched in sweat."

Ken punctuates his narrative with a favorite moral: *Never lie down in down and thermal with your clothes on.* Linda adds one of her own: "If you can survive a honeymoon like ours, you can survive anything."

If the story of Ken and Linda Aukett's honeymoon reveals anything, it's how well suited the two of them are for each other and defines their ability to survive. It's not only that they look alike—both wear thick, wide-rimmed glasses that highlight remarkably similar square-jawed chins that are softened by benign smiles and puckish eyes. It's also that they both suffered early in their lives from ulcerative colitis, leaving each of them with ileostomies. And they both share the same passion for helping other people with ostomies, volunteering their spare time serving the United Ostomy Association (UOA) and the International Ostomy Association (IOA), which is how they met. But that's yet another story.

It was 1981, the year of the infamous Air Traffic Controller's Strike. As the union leaders and President Reagan were locked nose to nose in a battle of wills, the airlines found themselves shorthanded, leaving many travelers stranded in airports throughout the country. Among those marooned in Buffalo, New York, one sweltering August day was thirty-eight-year-old Linda King, en route to a UOA conference in Minneapolis.

Linda, who had suffered from ulcerative colitis

since she was a teenager and had ostomy surgery when she was in her late twenties, became involved with the Ostomy Association almost immediately after her surgery in 1970. Beginning as State Representative in Upstate New York and progressing to Regional Coordinator for a large area that served most of New York, Ontario, and Quebec, she later served as Director of UOA's Regional Program. She also served three terms on the UOA Board of Directors and became National Secretary and then President before taking on additional responsibilities in the International Ostomy Association. She still chairs UOA's Committee for Government Affairs and attends each UOA Youth Rally as a counselor.

It was during her term as Regional Coordinator that she met Ken Aukett, who was also involved with the UOA, though his involvement had taken a more circuitous route. Like Linda, Ken had suffered from ulcerative colitis almost his entire life, but unlike Linda, whose disease was medically managed from the beginning, Ken never even discussed his problems with anyone. Symptoms would come and go, beginning when he was about eleven and recurring on and off throughout his high school and college years. He was finally diagnosed at age twenty-six, but—being a typical male, as he puts it—he put off dealing with the disease until it was almost too late.

In 1972, at the age of thirty-three, Ken was admitted to the emergency room while hemorrhaging from his large intestine. He awoke from surgery hours later with an ileostomy and acute peritonitis, which left him hospitalized for three months and near death's door. "You know it's serious," he reflects, "when your roommates in the hospital keep getting discharged, but you never do."

Ken's first contact with the UOA came while he was recovering in the hospital and the support organization sent him a visitor. All Ken remembers about the visit is that the guest was a little late (he had been playing tennis), and that the visitor told him he could now eat popcorn and drink beer ("What else is there?" Ken responded, chuckling). Though the visit was positive, Ken never sought additional help from the UOA, and he might never have gotten involved if it weren't for two watershed events that occurred in the aftermath of his surgery.

The first took place a few weeks after finally being discharged from the hospital. Ken had lost sixty pounds—"I didn't have a shadow," he says—and was still in the process of healing. The only way he could get comfortable was to sit on a rubber donut. In spite of this, Ken's surgeon asked him if he would mind returning to the hospital to visit with one of his patients about to undergo the same kind of surgery. "I went in there wearing a raincoat and looking like Ichabod Crane," Ken recalls. "I sat down gingerly on my rubber donut and said, 'I'm here to cheer you up.' The poor guy got up during that visit twice to use the bathroom. I think I scared the living daylights out of him."

The second watershed moment took place several years later. Ken picked up a copy of the *Philadelphia Inquirer* and happened upon an article profiling a South Jersey chapter of the United Ostomy Association. The story described a seventy-five-year-old woman from the UOA who was visiting a young man in the hospital. All well and good, but something about the story bothered Ken. "What was an older woman doing visiting a young man?" he thought. "Why isn't a young man visiting a young man?" It wasn't long before Ken's opinions turned into personal musings: "I should be doing this," he concluded.

Ken sought out the woman, who turned out to be the president of the local UOA chapter. He started asking questions, and within a year, he became actively involved in the organization. By the time he and Linda met that afternoon in August 1981, Ken was Regional Director of New Jersey and parts of New York, and well on his way to higher-profile posts within the UOA.

Though they knew of each other professionally, the two had never met personally—and their first meeting wouldn't necessarily qualify as a textbook-perfect first encounter. By then, Linda had just about had it. After her miserable layover in Buffalo, she managed to catch a flight out of western New York the following day and arrive in Minneapolis so late for the Board meeting that she decided to forgo checking into the hotel and instead make a mad dash for the conference room where the meeting was being held. Dragging her luggage behind her, she headed to the escalators and stepped onto the moving stairway. She began her ascent just fine, but behind her, lodged in the narrow passage of the escalator and going nowhere fast, was her luggage.

That was the proverbial last straw. By the time Linda reached the top, the meltdown was well underway. At that moment, Ken stepped into the hallway. There, at the top of the escalator, stood Linda, sobbing uncontrollably. He strode toward the damsel in distress, offered his assistance, and, he concluded gallantly, "I've been helping her ever since."

A Proposal

Well, sort of. It's not as though Linda is all that helpless. In fact, it was she, not he, who got them both on the dance floor at their annual banquet a year later, causing tongues to wag and heads to nod since you couldn't miss the couple. (Ken stands six feet, four inches tall, while Linda is five foot, nine inches.) "Ken doesn't usually dance at these affairs," explains Linda, who loves to dance. "In fact, he would usually turn the ladies down when they asked him." And it was she, not he, who got the ball rolling when it looked as if marriage were inevitable.

"It was around Christmas," Ken recalls, "and I had given Linda an aquamarine ring that my mother had worn. She put the ring on her right hand, but a couple days later, she turned to me and said, 'Now Ken, aren't we a bit old for friendship rings? Shouldn't I be moving it from my right hand to my left sometime soon?' I figured she must be proposing, so we got engaged."

Ken and Linda waited to finish their terms of office—he as president and she as secretary—before tying the knot in 1988. The wedding took place in a small church that Linda's parents attended in Romulus, New York. A reception in Seneca Falls followed the ceremony. There were about seventy guests in attendance, many of them from the Ostomy Association. It was the second marriage for both Ken and Linda and it was, says Ken, "one of the best weddings I've ever attended."

So, what's it like being a married couple with both partners having stomas?

The easy answer is that their ostomies have been a non-issue. On the practical side, the couple has adapted so well they joke about things like output and odors, and they can guess what each other had for breakfast or lunch by the gurgling sounds their stomas produce. The occasional accident or leak invariably finds its way into one of their lectures or workshops, and if either of them is ever in a pinch, they borrow each other's ostomy equipment. And as for equipment storage, the Auketts have even designed "His and Her" cabinets in the bathroom.

The fact that both Ken and Linda were in their late thirties and had developed a solid professional relationship as well as a good friendship before they married may account for the ease with which they entered this unusual pairing. "Neither of us had any problems accepting the fact that we were both ostomates," Linda replies. "By the time we got married, we knew each other so well that it was a natural progression from being involved professionally with the Association to being intimate with someone who also had an ostomy."

That said, both Ken and Linda acknowledge that just because a person has an ostomy is no guarantee he or she will be sympathetic to another person's ostomy. "Within the Association, we often encourage people to get involved with other ostomates—more for socialization than anything else," Ken explains. "If a person is single, this kind of socialization is vital. Nevertheless, you really don't know how accepting you are going to be, especially if a friendship evolves into romance. You would think there would be empathy, but it's no guarantee. Acceptance is not a given."

In Ken and Linda's case, neither of them was concerned about intimacy going into their relationship, and fortunately, neither was offended by the other's stoma.

Ken realizes that is not always the case. "Sometimes people have expectations that their partner will be perfect. Body image can be so important, and it can be a bit of a let-down if you're not prepared."

Ken and Linda are aware that this kind of surgery can be the last straw for some people. In their experience working with people with ostomies they have seen marriages fall apart after one of the partners had surgery. "It's been my experience that when a marriage is weak, the ostomy can be used as an excuse to break out of the relationship," explains Ken, who admits that his first marriage might have been adversely affected by his surgery. "Not only is it difficult for the non-ostomate spouse, but it's difficult for the person who has had the surgery. If you think back," he adds, "the very first thing you're rewarded for as a child is being potty trained. Now as an adult, you find yourself unable to control your bodily functions. Suddenly you feel unclean and out of control. It can be very difficult to accept."

The secret, says Ken, is finding something you both can get behind. For the Auketts, that something was their involvement with the Ostomy Association. "If one or the other of us didn't believe that giving our time to a cause like this was a good thing, our relationship probably wouldn't survive," he says. "We'd be like two people going down river rapids in a canoe trying to go different directions. If you can't agree, eventually you'll end up crashing on the rocks."

Ken, who since his honeymoon has braved several more canoeing trips with Linda, speaks from experience. He's had his share of arguing with his wife about which way to go before jamming up against rocks beneath the water's surface. Eventually, though, they managed to dislodge the canoe and get back on the river.

A metaphor, perhaps, for making a marriage work—ostomy or no ostomy.

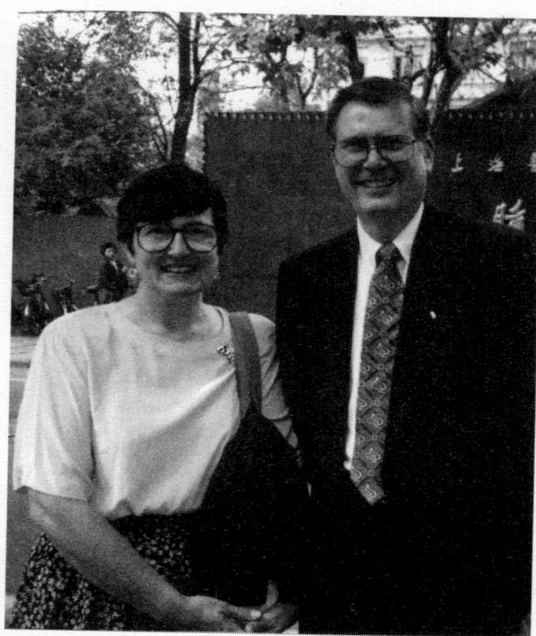

In a strange twist of fate, Ken and Linda Aukett each battled inflammatory disease and had ostomy surgery before meeting, falling in love, and getting married. Besides having the ability to finish each other's sentences, the Auketts really can say to each other, "I know what you're going through."

Each has lived with their ostomy for more than thirty years, and together they continue to camp and participate in other outdoors activities while donating their spare time to helping others through the United Ostomy Association.

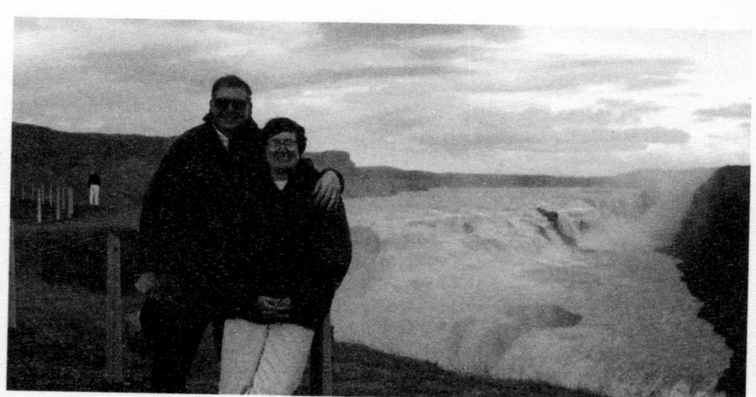

The Four Toughest Words

LOIS FINK

AGE
53

HOMETOWN
Edmonds, Washington

MEDICAL SITUATION
She started experiencing abdominal distress prior to puberty and suffered from Crohn's disease for nearly twenty years before needing a permanent ileostomy.

by Lois Fink

"You don't have appendicitis. You have Crohn's disease," the surgeon pronounced matter-of-factly, changing my life in one breath. I remember those four paralyzing words said to me thirty-six years ago as if they were yesterday.

I was seventeen years old and had been telling my parents and doctors for two years that something was terribly wrong with me, but no one would listen. My symptoms began in childhood. Stomach aches came and went, along with fevers that climbed quickly. At my cousin's Bar Mitzvah reception, the impatient photographer had no choice but to wait while I ran to the bathroom several times before he could take family photos. I was eleven years old and felt embarrassed and self-conscious.

A year later most of my female classmates were beginning to develop breasts. As for myself, I remained flat-chested and wondered when I would turn into a "woman." I prayed nightly to God for my first menstrual period, figuring if God could part the Red Sea when my ancestors fled Egypt, then God could certainly accomplish this minor miracle, yet it never happened. Still, I waited and waited, and my weight at the age of fourteen topped the scales between eighty and eighty-five pounds. By this time, my mother decided it was time for padded bras. I hated wearing them because they reminded me that I wasn't "normal," but the fear of not looking like my classmates overpowered my anger. Junior high gym class was an ordeal as I cringed in front of my locker while changing clothes. I wouldn't take a shower because I didn't want anybody to see my body.

Since my appetite was poor, my parents began bribing me with free use of their department store credit card if I would just get to ninety pounds. In the hands of most teenagers, that could spell financial disaster, but not in my case. I couldn't get to ninety pounds, and I didn't care about clothes. What good would they do me?

Shopping was always a nightmare. Clothes hung on me, and I didn't want to look in the mirror. "Look at you," my mother would say, "you are nothing but skin and bones." I hated myself and what I was becoming.

Visit After Visit

Meanwhile, the stomach aches and fevers continued and became more pronounced, along with the diarrhea. I was fifteen when the family physician prescribed Phenobarbital every six weeks for the "stomach flu" that seemed to visit my life regularly. When I turned sixteen, my mother, alarmed that there was still no sign of menstruation, took me to her gynecologist. Her main concern was whether I would be able to bear children. After the exam, the doctor assured my mother I could indeed have a family, but he was at a loss to explain why my ovaries weren't maturing.

The abdominal pain and diarrhea, which were intensifying and occurring with increasing regularity, began tormenting me at night as well as during the day. I was experiencing leg cramps caused by lack of potassium from the constant diarrhea.

My anxious mother, hoping to get an answer as to why I felt and looked the way I did, made the rounds from one doctor to another in my hometown of Pittsburgh, Pennsylvania. She was told there was nothing wrong with me. The leg cramps were a result of *growing pains!* Yet we couldn't see any signs of growth. Another doctor, after roughly administering a sigmoidoscopy, found nothing. He dismissed my symptoms, saying I was just nervous. "If you don't watch it," he warned, "you'll be a good candidate for colitis." Never mind that by this time, the abdominal pain was so intense that I nearly passed out on the way to class several times. I'd slump in the hallway and wait for the vice-like grip in my stomach to ease before I could walk again.

I vowed, after this visit, that I'd never see another physician. He and others were dismissive, uncompassionate, and so brutally rough when they examined me that I saw no reason to let another one near me.

After this last physician's "finding," my mother began to have talks with me. She'd explain that all the doctors said the same thing: there was nothing physically wrong with me, and I had to "get a grip" on myself. Otherwise, I would end up in a hospital—a mental hospital. After I assured my mother that I understood what she was trying to tell me, I went to my bedroom, where I stared into the mirror on my vanity. "There is nothing wrong with you, Lois," I repeated. "All the doctors have said so." The voice in my heart was saying something else. *There is something wrong. You're not making this up.*

The normal friction that results between mother and daughter during the volatile teen years was accentuated by my "phantom" illness. I didn't realize how frustrated and powerless my mother felt. The medical experts decreed there was nothing physically wrong with me, so it had to be "in my head." She was caught in the medical nightmare just as I was. The tension of wanting to believe me, while deferring to the medical experts, must have been unbearable for her.

Shortly after my seventeenth birthday, the symptoms intensified, and I began losing weight at an alarming rate. I was constantly thirsty, but the sight and smell of food nauseated me. This was my senior year in high school, the time for Homecoming and Prom and other memories that I was supposed to cherish. Because the mass was there and it "moved," I deduced that I had cancer since a moving mass equals cancer. A mass had developed in the lower left quadrant of my abdomen, which moved with every step I took. I made a detached self-diagnosis of cancer and calculated it was only a matter of time before I died.

Halfway through my senior year, I collapsed in excruciating pain. The initial diagnosis was appendicitis. My mother, stunned at these words, leveled her eyes at the family physician and said, "My daughter has been sick for nearly two years, and the medical profession is just now figuring this out?" His silent response was deafening. I was rushed to the hospital and prepped for an emergency appendectomy, which revealed not appendicitis, but an inflamed portion of the ileum—the last section of the small bowel. I had Crohn's disease, not appendicitis, but the surgeon was not able to proceed with an operation because of the severity of the inflammation. The surgeon closed me right back up. I was seventeen years old and weighed sixty-nine pounds, but at least now it was not all in my head.

I spent three weeks in the hospital, trying to come to grips with the diagnosis of Crohn's disease, feeling alone and isolated from my friends. To add insult to injury, I was not allowed to return to school; my health was deemed too precarious. I was home-schooled for the remaining four months of my senior year.

Shortly after this, my mother found a small magazine article about Suzanne Rosenthal, a New York woman who had been diagnosed with Crohn's disease. Her husband and friends were laying the groundwork for a foundation that would raise funds to find a cause and cure for Crohn's disease and ulcerative colitis. I carried that article in my purse for over a year. It was my only link with someone else who had gone through what I was going through. Knowing that someone else was out there helped me feel not quite so alone.

"Why me?" I angrily shouted at my father. Like my mother, Dad was feeling powerless at not being able to help his daughter, and he was clearly uncomfortable discussing this bowel disease with me. He tried to comfort me by suggesting, "Perhaps later in life you will be able to encourage someone else because of what you are now going through. You'll know what to say and how to help."

It would be years later, after coming to terms with this disease, that I began volunteering my time and energy to help others newly diagnosed with Crohn's disease or ulcerative colitis. Because I've been there, I know how to listen, and I can share my invaluable experience with others. My father's words not only proved true but also continue to inspire me and maintain a connection with him, even though he has passed away.

Treatment with Prednisone caused my body to swell with fluid, distorting my face. Swollen ankles made walking difficult. This steroid did increase my appetite, but I was put on a special diet that didn't allow much food at all. I was further isolated from my friends and couldn't go up to the local pizzeria with them. No French fries or Pepsi either!

Three months after my diagnosis, I was in the hospital again. This time, doctors were examining me, trying to figure out why my sexual development had been so delayed. I was poked, peered at, and discussed as if I weren't present. I felt like a bug under a microscope.

After five months on high doses of Prednisone, there was still no improvement, and surgery was recommended. My mother and I flew to Philadelphia to get a second opinion from one of the experts on Crohn's disease. He concurred that surgery was the only answer.

The night before I was to be admitted to the hospital was the night of my high school prom. As I sat outside on our front porch with my mother, I watched a neighbor friend step out in a beautiful formal gown, escorted by her father. While Mom expressed her sorrow that I wasn't going to the prom, I contemplated my upcoming surgery and uncertain future. The prom was the furthest thing from my mind. Crohn's disease had eclipsed everything around me.

Six inches of my small bowel and a foot-and-a-half of my large bowel were removed during that operation in 1966. The surgery was a success, and my recovery was rapid. For the first time in years, I enjoyed a normal life. I gained weight and began my freshman year at a local university. I also noticed that more information began appearing about Crohn's disease. I learned that if the disease is active during puberty, secondary growth and development can be delayed. Suddenly, the puzzle of my arrested physical development was solved.

My recovery was short-lived, however. Nearly one year to the day after my first bowel resection, fevers, diarrhea, and weight loss returned. I landed in the hospital again, and college came to a halt. Then began a regimen that would continue for years: high doses of steroids, minimum attendance at college, and limited food choices. Slowly, ever so slowly, I was able to decrease the steroids until at last I resembled myself when I looked in a mirror. I still could only take three classes a semester in college, but the days when I'd be so depressed that I'd cry for hours seemed to be fading. The inflammation was gradually calming, and I'll never forget the wonderful day that I ate a juicy, fresh peach!

I led a fairly normal life for about eight years. I still went to the bathroom three or four times a day, but I could live with that. But in 1975, things changed rapidly. I was rushed to the emergency room with a small bowel obstruction. I'd been experiencing intense abdominal pain for a week, and everyone at work was telling me it was stress-induced. I knew better. If the surgery, which was performed several days later, had been delayed much longer, my bowel would have perforated. Once again, the same routine: high doses of steroids and limited food choices. I knew this by heart.

As the disease progressed into the large bowel and became more advanced, my life gradually changed to accommodate it. I had to know the exact location of a bathroom wherever I went. Close friends joked that I knew where all the bathrooms were in town. On a flight to Los Angeles, I was headed down the aisle to the bathroom when the "fasten your seatbelt" sign flashed. The stewardess blocked my way. I told her in no uncertain terms that the turbulence going on inside me was far worse than what was happening outside. She stepped aside.

At a party, I was always aware if the bathroom was occupied. If it was, I became uneasy. A leisurely walk in the park or an extended car trip was a source of extreme anxiety. I could never sit through a movie or enjoy a restaurant meal without using the ladies room at least once. If I went shopping for clothes, I'd check to see whether the fitting rooms were in close proximity to the bathroom. There were days when I'd be completely "bathroom bound." I couldn't leave the house because I constantly had to use the toilet.

I'd be up several times a night, as well. I took medication to slow the motility of the GI track, but I was fighting a losing battle. When the entire colon and rectum were diseased, I experienced the humiliation of losing control. I was mortified. I learned to carry spare underwear and pantyhose. I stopped wearing shorts. At least if I had an accident, things weren't so noticeable if I were wearing blue jeans. One day while shopping, I couldn't get to the bathroom in time and lost control. Fighting the tears, I hurried to my car hoping nobody would know what had just happened. It seemed to take forever to get home and even longer to feel clean.

Only a few longtime friends knew what I was going through; I was too humiliated and afraid of what people might think. My disease and losing control were my secrets, which is why the prospect of dating terrified me. "How can I possibly share this with a man? How will he understand?" I tearfully asked my closest friend. I agreed to a few dates, but I never wanted to take a budding relationship to the next level. In an effort to find some humor in what I was going through, I'd joke about my worst nightmare: having to arm-wrestle an eighty-year-old woman for a vacant bathroom stall! The walls of my life gradually closed in until the only place I felt secure was in my house and in my bathroom.

When I was thirty-six years old, I had no choice but to concede to the inevitable. Bowel resections—the surgical removal of a diseased portion of intestine and joining together the remaining ends of bowel to restore intestinal continuity—were no longer an option. Now, my doctor told me, I had to consider undergoing a proctocolectomy and permanent ileostomy. In other words, doctors would surgically remove the colon and rectum and bring the end of the small bowel through the abdominal wall, allowing drainage of intestinal waste.

Fecal material would be collected in a small appliance or "bag" that covered the end of the bowel or stoma, which is usually located on the right lower abdomen just below the belt line. Ever since I'd been diagnosed with inflammatory bowel disease, this type of operation had been my nightmare. Now it was threatening to become a reality. "I won't have that surgery," I declared to my doctor. "I won't be mutilated." He shrugged his shoulders and wished me the best, but two years later, I was back. I had no choice. As terrified as I was, I knew I had to have this operation.

My doctor introduced me to another patient who had gone through this surgery the previous year, and she became my "mentor." The first time we met, she wore a skintight jumpsuit, and I remember staring at her in astonishment. I thought I'd have to have a completely different wardrobe to hide the appliance. She smiled and sat through the entire two-hour meeting without using the bathroom. Now that made an impression on me. My "homework" was to list on paper what I hated about having Crohn's disease and why I wanted this operation. I came up with fifteen reasons. When I wrote, "I'm tired of being an observer of life and not an active participant," I knew I was ready.

With this woman's support and a volunteer with the local chapter of the Crohn's and Colitis Foundation of America (CCFA), I was emotionally prepared for the surgery that would change my life for the better. The fear that I wouldn't like myself after this body-altering surgery didn't materialize. What I experienced was freedom for the first time in nineteen years: freedom to walk in the park, enjoy a trip, watch a movie, or enjoy a meal, all without interruption because I needed to go to the bathroom. Freedom to listen to someone when they were talking to me instead of worrying if my body would betray or embarrass me.

Our society is uneasy about discussing bathroom

habits as well as the part of the body that deals with elimination. We are taught it isn't acceptable to discuss diarrhea in "polite company." We use euphemisms to describe what goes on in the bathroom, and we are squeamish or laugh nervously when talking about problems "below the belt." Emotional healing begins when feelings can be openly shared.

Sixteen years after my ileostomy, I've made peace with Crohn's disease. Gone are the days when I'd be in such denial that I would rebel by not taking my medication. Gone are the days when I was too embarrassed or afraid to discuss what was happening to my body.

Gone are the days when I lived life wondering where the closest bathroom was. I have a lot to live for and a lot to be thankful for. I wonder what life would have been like if I had my ostomy surgery earlier. My surgery gave back what Crohn's disease took away—my life.

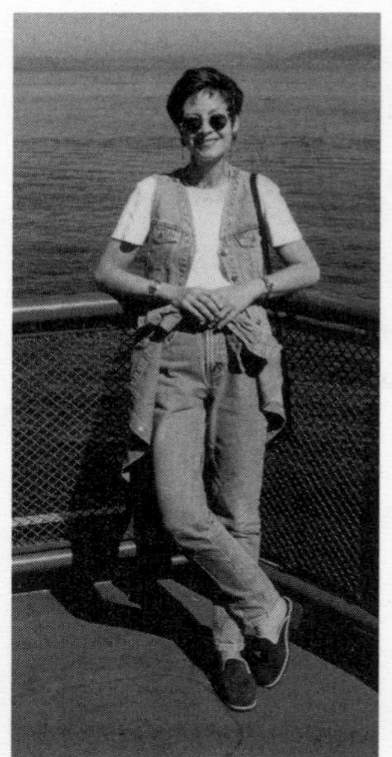

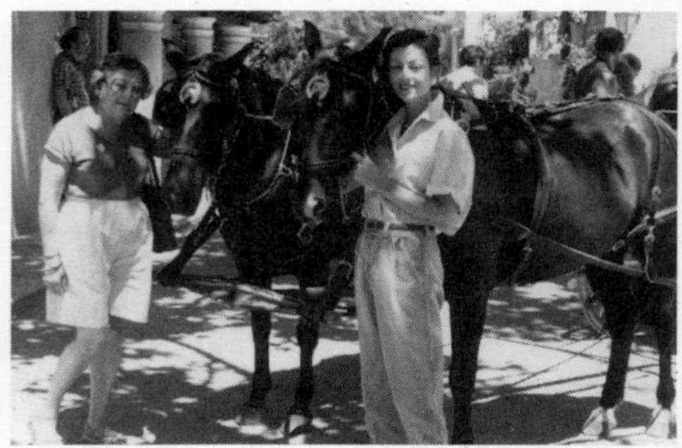

When Lois Fink was growing up, she kept trying to tell people that something was wrong. She looked anorexic and at one point, weighed just over ninety pounds. Mercifully, the doctors determined it was not just "in her head" and diagnosed her condition as Crohn's disease. It wasn't until her mid-thirties, however, when a permanent ileostomy changed life for the better. These days, Lois loves to travel. She's pictured above with her mother, Anna, in Sedona, Arizona.

OSTOMY INFORMATION

Living With an Ostomy

When first considering ostomy surgery, many people are concerned that the operation will dramatically alter their lives. Though any surgery should be considered carefully, an ostomy can be the key that opens the door to opportunities locked away by illness. For people who have ulcerative colitis, this operation offers a cure. The following are questions that are most commonly asked by people who are considering ostomy surgery.

What is an ostomy?

There are various types of ostomy surgery, depending on the nature of the illness. A common option for ulcerative colitis is the creation of an ileostomy. The entire colon and, in some cases, the rectum are removed in a one or two-step procedure. The surgeon creates an opening in the abdominal wall, through which the ileum is rerouted to the outside, creating a stoma. To collect stool as it exits the ileum, a disposable pouch is attached to the skin around the stoma with medical adhesive. Since a permanent ostomy is not a cure for Crohn's disease, it is performed only when the disease cannot be controlled medically. Some conditions (e.g., a bowel perforation or abscess) may require a temporary ostomy.

How much time must I allow for daily care?

The maintenance of an ostomy requires only minor

modifications in your routine. Daily care consists of emptying the pouch when it becomes one-third to one-half full. You can do this in any bathroom, private or public. This process requires no additional equipment and takes little more time than you previously required to "go to the bathroom." In fact, it may be less time-consuming, especially if diarrhea plagued you before surgery.

Ostomy pouches, like your rectum, have a finite capacity and will overflow or leak if they become too full. Most people report that they need to empty the pouch four to six times a day. You should note the occasions when the stoma is more active (e.g., after meals), and set aside time to empty your pouch. To avoid interrupting sleep, it is helpful to drain the pouch at bedtime, but you may want to empty it again should a full bladder awaken you.

What kinds of pouching systems are available?

Ostomy "appliances" are designed to meet individual needs. There are one-and two-piece systems, pouches with built-in skin barriers, drainable and closed-end pouches, styles offering various depth of convexity, pouches with built-in gas relief valves and filters, and combinations of these features. Years ago, certain types of pouches were designated for specific surgeries (e.g., an ileostomy required a drainable pouching system). Though more options are available today, some ostomies are more difficult to manage than others and require recommendations by healthcare professionals.

How can I find the system that is best for me?

You may want to consult an enterostomal therapy

nurse (ETN), a registered nurse who specializes in ostomy care. The ETN will recommend a pouching system and will teach you how to care for the stoma. After your discharge from the hospital, she is available for follow-up care. In time, your pouching needs may change, as normal post-operative stomal swelling diminishes or your weight changes. As your self-reliance grows, you can work with your ETN to select a new system.

How do I care for the skin around the stoma?

Proper attention to the skin around an ileostomy can eliminate painful bouts of raw or reddened skin. Known as "stomal effluent," the stool from an ileostomy usually is liquid and contains enzymes and other digestive acids native to the small intestine. These materials break down the proteins in food, making them easier to absorb. The enzymes, however, cannot distinguish between the proteins they attack and your skin. Thus, if the stomal effluent remains in contact with the skin for too long, painful irritation can result.

People who have ileostomies should never patch a leaking pouch with tape. Change the entire system, and be sure to clean the skin first. Burning or itching under the pouch indicates that some stomal effluent has leaked onto the skin. Pectin-based or hydrocolloid skin barriers always should be used for ileostomy management. They may be used in conjunction with a skin barrier paste. Avoid harsh soaps when cleaning this area. The opening in the pouching system should be accurately sized to prevent the possibility of stool leakage.

Will I require a special diet?

If a particular food bothered you before surgery, it probably will continue to do so. For example, if you suffered from lactose intolerance before surgery, dairy products sill may cause diarrhea, bloating, and gas. Some people find, however, that they are able to eat foods that they could not tolerate before.

You may need to avoid high residue or "stringy" foods, such as popcorn and peanuts, because they can cause blockages in the bowel. Don't worry if seeds from cucumbers, tomatoes, or fruits appear whole in your pouch. Even an intact intestinal system will not digest these foods.

If you are unsure about a particular food, try a small portion. If you have no problems, you might try a larger portion next time. Remember, also, that taking time to chew food thoroughly will improve digestion.

People who have ileostomies need to maintain a fluid intake of eight to ten glasses a day or more. To replace potassium and sodium lost in ileostomy effluent, drink such fluids as tea and tomato or fruit juices, in addition to water. Sport drinks such as Gatorade are also excellent for replacing vital electrolytes.

Will the stool in my pouch cause odor?

With proper care, odor need not be a concern. Indeed, you probably have met someone with an ostomy and were unaware of his condition. (Up to 1 million people in North America have ostomies!)

To combat odor, avoid foods that cause gas. You may also use products specifically designed to control pouch odor:

• Pouch deodorizers. These commercially available products, usually liquids, are placed inside the pouch each time it is emptied. The most effective agents attack the odor-causing bacteria, rather than simply mask odor.

• Internal agents, such as chlorophyll tablets or bismuth subgallate. These over-the-counter products are taken orally several times a day, or with meals.

• Room deodorizers. One spray of a concentrated ostomy deodorizer can freshen the air after you empty your pouch.

Can I have a normal sexual relationship?

It's natural to be concerned that an ostomy may alter your ability to function sexually, to feel desirable, and to be the recipient of another's love. But many people find that their sex life improves after ostomy surgery.

Your ability to feel attractive and "sexy" comes from feeling good about yourself. When you are ill, your sex drive may decrease. Perceiving ostomy surgery as a release from illness can help you return to healthy sexual functioning.

In general, an ostomy's impact on your sex life is related to your mind, not your body. Occasionally, however, surgical removal of the rectum can affect a male's ability to have an erection. But this is the exception, not the rule. When careful excision of the rectum is performed, most males retain their ability to have and to maintain an erection.

Discussing your concerns about sexuality with your surgeon or ETN, both before and after surgery, will help you through the initial adjustment period.

Will ostomy surgery affect my ability to have children?

An ostomy provides no barriers to a woman's ability to become pregnant or to have a healthy baby. The only inconvenience may be changes in stomal contour and size during pregnancy, due to increases in abdominal girth. These changes are easily managed by accommodating the pouching system to the fluctuations of the stoma size and shape. A vaginal birth is possible, unless your obstetrician recommends a caesarean section. It's important that your obstetrician consult your surgeon during your pregnancy.

Will an ostomy restrict my physical activity?

Activities, such as jogging, skiing, aerobic exercise, swimming, and even rollerblading, are not contraindicated because of an ostomy. But you will have to avoid vigorous contact sports and heavy lifting. For example, playing football can injure the intestinal tissue from which the stoma is created. Lifting anything heavier than twenty-five pounds can increase intra-abdominal pressure, which can lead to further complications, such as parastomal hernia. This does not mean, however, that you cannot pick up your baby! If work demands heavy lifting or some other strenuous activity, discuss this situation with your surgeon and your employer. Indeed, if you're in doubt about any activity, consult your physician.

Remember, ostomy surgery can give you a new lease on life. Enjoy it!

GWEN B. TURNBULL, R.N., B. SED, C.E.T.N.

Facts About Inflammatory Bowel Disease

• Crohn's disease and ulcerative colitis (collectively known as inflammatory bowel disease, or IBD, because their symptoms and complications are similar) are chronic digestive disorders of the small and large intestines.

• It is estimated that two million Americans suffer from IBD, with 30,000 new cases diagnosed in the U.S. each year. New cases per day average 82, or 3.5 an hour.

• Anyone can get IBD, but young adults between the ages of 20 and 40 are most susceptible. (Ten percent, or 200,000, of those afflicted are youngsters under the age of 18.)

• Symptoms range from mild to severe and life-threatening and include any or all of the following:

persistent diarrhea
abdominal pain or cramps
blood passing through the rectum
fever and weight loss
skin or eye irritations
delayed growth and retarded sexual maturation in children

• Approximately 20 percent of patients have another family member with IBD, although a specific genetic pattern has not been identified.

• Both the cause of and cure for IBD are unknown.

TREATMENT

• Medications currently available alleviate inflammation and reduce symptoms but do not provide a cure. The principle drugs used to treat both Crohn's disease and ulcerative colitis are sulvasalazine and corticosteroids.

• A number of new medications, derivatives of corticosteroids and sulfasalazine, are currently awaiting FDA approval. Four such drugs, Asacol®, Rowasa®, Dipentum®, and Pentasa®, have been approved since 1988. Remicade has also been shown to be effective in many patients with Crohn's disease.

• Immunosuppressive agents, such as azathioprine (Imuran®) and 6-murcaptopurine (6-MP), are other medications used to treat IBD, especially in persons who do not respond to more standard treatments.

• IBD is an unpredictable illness—some patients recover after a single attack or are in remission for years; others require frequent hospitalizations and even surgery. Symptoms may vary in nature, frequency, and intensity.

• Without proper treatment, symptoms may worsen considerably and complications may occur.

• Colon cancer may be a serious complication of long-term ulcerative colitis involving the whole colon, even in a patient who is in remission.

SURGERY

• Surgery is sometimes recommended when medication can no longer control the symptoms, when there are intestinal obstructions, or when other complications arise.

• An estimated two-thirds to three-quarters of persons with Crohn's disease will have one or more operations in the course of their lifetime. The surgery for Crohn's disease, however, is not considered a permanent cure, because the disease frequently returns elsewhere in the gastrointestinal tract. For ulcerative colitis, surgical removal of the entire colon and rectum (colectomy) is a permanent cure. Approximately 25-40 percent of ulcerative colitis patients will require surgery at some point during their illness.

EMOTIONAL FACTORS

• IBD is not a psychosomatic illness—there is no evidence to suggest that emotions play a causative role. IBD flare-ups may occur, however, during times of emotional or physical stress.

DIET

• There is no link between eating certain kinds of foods and IBD, but dietary modifications, especially during severe flare-ups, can help reduce disease symptoms and replace lost nutrients.

EFFECTS ON THE PERSON WITH IBD

• The economic and social burden on patients and their families can be enormous. Children and adults must interrupt school and work for repeated hospital stays, and medical and disability insurance often are unavailable.

The Ten Most Common Myths About Crohn's Disease and Ulcerative Colitis

MYTH 1: Crohn's disease and ulcerative colitis are caused by stress.

There is no evidence that Crohn's disease and ulcerative colitis are caused by stress. But, as with any chronic illness, symptoms may worsen during a particularly stressful period in a person's life.

MYTH 2: Certain personality types are more prone to develop ulcerative colitis or Crohn's disease.

IBD sufferers were once perceived as people who were emotional or nervous. However, a study conducted by Johns Hopkins University and Medical School concluded that the personality profile of people with IBD does not differ significantly from that of healthy persons.

MYTH 3: Crohn's disease and ulcerative colitis affect primarily older adults.

Anyone can get IBD, but young adults between the ages of 20 and 40 are most susceptible. (Ten percent, or 200,000, of those afflicted are youngsters under the age of 18.) It is estimated that only 5 to 15 percent of IBD patients develop the disease later in life.

MYTH 4: Symptoms can be controlled through diet.

There is no evidence that diet causes IBD. Most people can tolerate a normal diet. In some cases, however, dietary restrictions must be imposed. Some IBD sufferers find that the lactose in milk causes cramps, pain, gas and diarrhea. Others find a low-fiber diet (avoiding such foods as fruit, vegetables, nuts, bran and whole grains) helps control symptoms.

MYTH 5: Crohn's disease and ulcerative colitis are "Jewish diseases."

It's true that individuals of Jewish ancestry are two to three times more likely to develop IBD. But researchers know that IBD does not discriminate. Crohn's disease and ulcerative colitis affect persons from every ethnic and racial group, men and women equally.

MYTH 6: African-Americans don't get IBD.

IBD has always been considered more common in whites. However, recent studies show a rising trend among black women.

MYTH 7: Individuals with ulcerative colitis will eventually develop colon cancer.

Under 5 percent of ulcerative colitis patients develop colon cancer. These usually are persons who have had the disease for ten years or more. As a preventative measure, gastroenterologists recommend that patients have a colonoscopy every two years. This exam allows the physician to spot cancer or precancerous changes within the colon.

MYTH 8: Women with IBD have difficulty becoming pregnant.

Women with IBD whose symptoms are under control get pregnant just as easily as women in the general population. Women with active Crohn's disease, however, may have difficulty becoming pregnant until their symptoms are brought under control.

MYTH 9: Many IBD sufferers end up on disability.

While disability may be the only solution in particularly severe cases, most people are able to work and lead productive lives. Indeed, people with IBD are employed in all areas of business and government, at every level.

MYTH 10: People with Crohn's disease and ulcerative colitis cannot live active lives.

Doctors encourage persons with IBD to follow a normal routine. Most people live fulfilling, active lives: they work, raise families, have healthy sex lives, and exercise regularly.

About the Authors

Rolf Benirschke, a former placekicker, played his ntire ten-year career with the San Diego Chargers from 977-86. He retired with sixteen team records and as the hird-most accurate kicker in NFL history. He received umerous awards during his career, including NFL Man f the Year and Comeback Player of the Year. He was lso named to the NFL All-Pro team during his playing ays, and following his retirement, he was inducted into ne Chargers Hall of Fame. Today, he is a noted speaker nd author and continues his involvement in several usinesses in San Diego.

Rolf also remains active with many different charible organizations in the San Diego community, includng Scripps Hospital, the United Way, the San Diego oo, as well as serving as a National Trustee for the rohn's & Colitis Foundation of America (CCFA). He is lso a longtime supporter of the United Ostomy ssociation and acts as a spokesman for ConvaTec, a ristol-Myers Squibb company, and Intermune, a iotech company active in the fight against hepatitis C.

Rolf and his wife, Mary, recently celebrated their velfth wedding anniversary and are the proud parents of our children: Erik, Kari, Tim, and Ryan. They continue to eside in the San Diego area.

Elaine Minamide, a writer living in Escondido, alifornia, has written for numerous newspapers and magzines. Also providing editorial assistance was Mike orkey, who collaborated with Rolf on his first book, *Alive Kicking*, which has more than 60,000 copies in print.

Looking for a Powerful Motivational Speaker?

Consider bringing Rolf Benirschke and his remarkable story of faith and courage as he shares what it took to come back from a near fatal illness and four major abdominal surgeries to play again in the National Football League.

Rolf has been inspiring audiences for more than twenty years. Groups like Elan Pharmaceutical, Tyco Healthcare, Toshiba, The Hartford, Baxter, Bristol-Myers Squibb, and many others have benefited from his moving presentations.

To learn more about his speaking availability please call toll-free (800) 560-9700 or (858) 552-4427 You can reach him via the Internet at:

www.greatcomebacks.com

Would You Like to Purchase Extra Copies of This Book?

If you would like to purchase additional copies of *Great Comebacks from Ostomy Surgery* or Rolf's first book, *Alive & Kicking*, copies are available for $16.95 plus shipping and handling. Quantity discounts are available. To contact Rolf please write:

Rolf Benirschke Enterprises
P.O. Box 9922
Rancho Santa Fe, CA 92067
(800) 560-9700
(858) 552-4427

Audiotape Series

Also available is an audiocassette series entitled "You're Not Alone," featuring Rolf's candid discussions about ostomy surgery with Marvin Bush (President George Bush's son), Al Geiberger (Senior PGA golfer), Suzanne Rosenthal (who helped found the Crohn's & Colitis Foundation of America), and Tip O'Neill (former U.S. Speaker of the House). The cost for this two-cassette series is $22.95 and can be ordered by contacting us at:

Rolf Benirschke Enterprises
P.O. Box 9922
Rancho Santa Fe, CA 92067
(800) 560-9700
(858) 552-4427